Resilient Health

Resilient Health

How to Thrive in Our Toxic World

Valencia Porter, MD, MPH

RESILIENT HEALTH: HOW TO THRIVE IN OUR TOXIC WORLD

Published by Enlighten Health Media

To my mother, who always encouraged me to pursue my studies and to persevere through any challenge or obstacle. She was the first one to teach me about the healing power of foods and to appreciate the wonders of nature. Later, her illnesses (and my similarity to her) fueled me to look beyond the standard of care, to keep asking why, and to search for what could be done to prevent and reverse disease. I feel her presence in every pot of nurturing food, in every flower, and in every warm hug.

Praise for Resilient Health

It's such a challenge to live in this modern-day world, inundated by toxins that we can't tolerate or avoid. We are exposed and vulnerable. And yet there is hope, because Dr. Valencia Porter's *Resilient Health* is exactly the book we all need right now! Arm yourself and your family with this valuable information, implement Dr. Porter's suggested practices- and you will strengthen your resilience. *Resilient Health* should be in every home - and used for reference again and again!

-Lissa Coffey, author of *The Perfect Balance Diet*, founder of CoffeyTalk.com

Dr. Valencia Porter is a magnificent expression of a modern-day integrative healer - blending her vast expertise in neurology, nutrition, and mind-body healing with her sheer genius in environmental science. In *Resilient Health*, Dr. Porter helps us navigate through the toxic world around us bringing us back to our innate wholeness. In the process, we heal, strengthen, and learn to thrive!

-davidji, author of *Sacred Powers*

If you have been wondering why you just cannot get well, Dr. Valencia Porter might have the answer. Environmental toxins that are highly prevalent, yet invisible, may be at the root of what ails you. In *Resilient Health*, Dr Porter provides straight-forward ways to identify sources of toxins and strengthen your body's detoxification systems. Follow her guidance to detoxify your body and home leading you to robust health!

-Victoria Maizes, MD, author of *Be Fruitful: The Essential Guide to Maximizing Fertility and Giving Birth to a Healthy Child*

Dr Porter is an early visionary who grasped the fact that the majority of diseases are caused, to some degree, by pollutants in our everyday environmental. Her book provides great insight into this truth and gives easy-to-follow guidance that will guide a multitude of fortunate readers into greater health and wellbeing.

-Walter J. Crinnion, ND, author of *Clean, Green & Lean*

Dr. Valencia Porter has created an astounding book—a truly holistic approach to eliminating toxins—internally and exter-nally. Steeped in science, *Resilient Health* offers easily acces-sible in-depth information and fascinating case studies from her own practice. She addresses this puzzle by addressing food sensitivities, unique body types known as doshas, and beneficial microbes. She also explores in detail how different environments impact us and offers solid solutions from: how to access healthful water, creating green home and garden-ing practices, to how electronic devices effect us. Last but not least she explores how our emotions and state of mind also can create a toxic or uplifting influence offering solutions for all.

- Candice Covington, author of *Essential Oils in Spiritual Practice: Working with the Chakras, Divine Archetypes, and the Five Great Elements*

Resilience is the ability to maintain homeostasis in the face of environmental setbacks. Dr. Valencia Porter is a renowned integrative physician who is an authority on facilitating vibrant health. *Resilient Health* is an authoritative guide to promoting optimum health and well-being by averting and mitigating toxic exposures by awareness, assessment, and action.

-Gerard E. Mullin, MD, author of *The Gut Balance Revolution*

Resilient Health is an excellent handbook for detoxification and rejuvenation. Dr. Porter effectively communicates the need to purify your diet & lifestyle to prevent the onslaught of many chronic diseases.

-Dr. Suhas Kshirsagar BAMS, MD (Ayurveda), author of *Hot Belly Diet* and *Change Your Schedule Change Your Life*

Table of Contents

Foreword by Deepak Chopra, M.D.

I'd like to give a context to this beneficial, expertly written, and heartfelt book. Being healthy has gone through different phases without people paying much attention to how radically things can shift. In our lifetime, to say "I'm healthy" once meant a state of ignorance about medical matters including even the most basic prevention. Health was a given, and its opposite was disease, something a doctor took care of. Then came the phase where "I'm healthy" took prevention into account, and campaigns against cholesterol and tobacco, for instance, shifted more responsibility on to the patient, away from total dependence on doctors.

But telling people to take responsibility for themselves doesn't mean that they will—prevention ran into one major obstacle: noncompliance. Millions of people said "I'm healthy" when what they meant was "I know what's good for me, but I haven't gotten around to doing it." Non-compliance led to the current situation where obesity, chronic disorders like type 2 diabetes, hypertension, and heart disease, along with certain cancers, are a paradox. They are largely preventable but epidemic at the same time. The missing element was self-awareness.

Dr. Valencia Porter stands on the cusp of the next wave, where "I'm healthy" means "I'm aware of what should be done, and I am willing to take care of myself." This attitude takes more words to express, but it simply links self-awareness with self-care. Once you value yourself, you automatically feel the desire to take care of yourself. Prevention was based on information; self-care is based on consciousness—in other words, on waking up.

Waking up to your own wellness begins a lifelong journey of discovery. One eye-opening aspect of Dr. Porter's book is to show us how much we take for granted and how little we know. In my generation of medical students in the late Sixties, very little was taught about prevention, and fields that Dr. Porter is completely trained in were unknown, including environmental medicine and integrative medicine. In med school we memorized hundreds of new terms; "holistic" wasn't one of them.

Resilient Health is a title that sends a message—we need to evolve in our approach to health and take heed of a medical revolution at the same time. This is one of the most exciting promises of this book, that the body's miraculous and mysterious healing system, about which too little is still known, can evolve. Moreover, this evolution is a matter of conscious choice. No longer is it true, as previous generations accepted, that biology is destiny. As every page you are about to read illustrates, biology is opportunity instead.

Readers will also appreciate that Dr. Porter's approach, while taking a sweeping and knowledgeable view of pollutants and toxins at every level of life, isn't dire or fear-based. Fear is a poor motivator in the long run, while inspiration and hope are excellent motivators for a lifetime. The knowledge about detoxification offered here opens up many pathways to purification, and taking any one of them, even with small steps, brings true personal growth. "I'm healthy" is coming to mean something no one imagined even twenty or thirty years ago: "I'm the wave of the future, a conscious being who will only be fulfilled when I am in tune with my body, my surroundings, the planet, and Nature as a whole." Such a goal implies an audacious agenda for future generations. But when the goal is laid out with Valencia Porter's remarkable range of knowledge, the wellness movement becomes a joyful project.

Introduction

"It ain't what you don't know that gets you into trouble. It's what you know for sure that just ain't so."

- Mark Twain

We live in an amazing time for medicine, health, and wellness. Technological advances, expansion of knowledge, and global connectivity have allowed for a vast array of innovative tools for the diagnosis, management, and treatment of disease. But despite state-of-the-art medical technology and an ever-increasing array of pharmaceutical medications, more than half of Americans are chronically ill, and many diseases are on the rise, such as obesity, autism, autoimmune diseases, asthma, allergies, infertility, certain cancers (liver, kidney, melanoma), and some infectious diseases. Chronic diseases are responsible for 70 percent of deaths each year and account for 86 percent of US health care costs, and it is quite common to have multiple chronic diseases or conditions at the same time—accounting for the vast majority of health care utilization and spending. Illnesses such as diabetes and cancer are reaching epidemic proportions, even in young people. And for the first time, a new generation is not expected to live longer than their parents. The modern medical approach focusing on diagnosis, management, and treatment of illness is certainly of value, particularly in acute, life-threatening conditions such as trauma. But with so many of these chronic diseases largely preventable, why are we waiting to act only once an illness has manifested? Isn't it better to try to keep the train on the tracks instead of making a massive effort to right it once it's gone off the rails and created collateral damage? How can we be resilient and thrive in our increasingly busy and toxic world?

As a medical student at the University of Southern California, I remember being frustrated by practicing what I felt was Band-Aid medicine. I kept seeing the same patients with the same problems, patching them up only to send them back out to resume their same old habits and actions, with little support, and no plan to address their underlying problems. Often, they wound up back in the ER as so-called "frequent flyers." I recall after a particularly difficult night caring for a homeless patient with alcohol withdrawal, I felt ineffective as a healer. Sure, we had probably saved his life, but what was the course for the remainder of his days? I could see that without treating his core issues, his future was most likely grim. I was disheartened. I had gone into medicine because I wanted to make a difference. Not just to keep people breathing and with a pulse, but to live optimal and vibrant lives.

Experiences like this eventually led me to study Preventive Medicine at the University of California San Diego. Not only did I want to treat people when they were sick, I wanted to know how to keep people healthy and well and how to empower them to take charge of their own health. I wanted to help keep the train on its tracks to prevent the train wreck and to know the best ways to get it back to functioning if it did happen to get derailed. I wanted to give my patients the option of an ounce of prevention instead of a pound of cure.

From acupuncture to Ayurveda, from herbs to homeopathy, from nutrition to mind-body techniques, and from environ-mental health to functional medicine, my interests led me to study a wide-range of healing modalities and ultimately become one of the first physicians to be board certified in Integrative Medicine. A burgeoning field, Integrative Medicine takes into account the whole person, emphasizes the therapeutic relationship between patient and practitioner, and allows for use of all appropriate therapies. I am blessed to be able to combine all of this in my private practice and at the Chopra Center for Wellbeing, where I see patients from around the world. Together, we look at all aspects of their lives to create a personalized holistic plan for wellness. For many patients, however, I discovered that in order to restart their body's natural ability to heal, we needed to manage their exposure to toxins in the environment and help them to detoxify; this is often a missing link to getting healthy and staying healthy. By addressing this root cause of illness, I have seen profound impacts on even chronic and "unexplained" conditions.

It took me many years to fully recognize the importance of the interaction between our health and the environment and the potential benefits of supporting and enhancing our ability to detoxify. Although this might make sense to you, you might be surprised to know that this is not part of conventional medical thinking. In medical school, we learned that the liver and kidneys were our primary detoxification organs and there was nothing more to it—unless you had a problem with one of those major organs or an acute poisoning. Then, and only then, you might need lifesaving treatment in a hospital because an inability to clear toxins—even those produced by our body's natural metabolic processes—can lead to dire consequences. For everyday purposes, however, our bodies were well designed to handle most toxic exposures without additional support. Or so I was told.

But what if our toxic load has drastically increased in the last century? What if our bodies now have to handle an additional 84,000 man-made chemicals and electromagnetic fields that didn't exist before in our environment? What if some of these chemicals were designed to remain in the environment and were never studied to determine if they were safe to use? What if the food that we eat is laced with chemicals that make us fat, sick, and tired and stripped of nutrients that support detoxification and promote health? What if the water that we drink is contaminated with heavy metals, pharmaceutical drugs, and chemicals that are toxic to our nervous, hormonal, and immune systems? What if the air that we breathe outside is polluted, and the air inside our homes and offices is even worse? What if we are now leading more stressful, busy lives on less sleep? What if we have become genetically less able to process toxins? Could our bodies still handle the load? Or is environmental toxicity the fly in the ointment that is keeping people from being well and able to thrive?

Having spent more than a decade researching how environmental toxins affect human health, I know one thing for sure: Everybody on the planet is burdened by a toxic load. Humans have always had to handle toxins from metabolic waste products, breakdown of bacteria in our body, heavy metals in our environment, combustion by-products from fires, including those used for cooking, and ingestion of naturally-occurring toxins, such as aflatoxin from moldy foods. But in today's world, we face a new barrage of man-made chemicals and pollutants that add to our burden. An ever-increasing number of chemicals are being released into the environment, and although they may be useful, many of them accumulate in the environment, build up in our bodies, and overwhelm our natural detoxification systems. Many of these toxins are known to affect our hormones, our nervous system, our immune function, and more, causing our bodies to get out of balance—or worse, become ill. Now more than ever, we need help to handle our toxic load.

When we manage our toxic load by reducing everyday toxic exposures and enhancing the body's ability to detoxify, the body is less stressed and therefore able to work better. We become more resilient. Our health-promoting genes are turned on and disease-promoting genes are turned off. As a result, the body is able to heal—preventing and reversing illness—and we are able to thrive. I have witnessed the amazing power of detoxification practices with my patients and in myself. While it can take time to get the body back on track, I have seen miraculous recoveries in some patients even after a short period of cleansing and rejuvenation: a patient diagnosed with multiple sclerosis who came to the clinic in a wheelchair and six days later literally walked out the door; many patients with long-term chronic fatigue who finally felt better; many patients with fibromyalgia or chronic pain conditions who became pain-free or pretty darn close; patients with insomnia who could finally sleep through the night; patients with skin conditions which drastically improved; and the list goes on. Most of these patients had sought help for months, or even years, consulting with multiple doctors and trying a variety of pharmaceutical medications and other treatments. It was only after addressing the whole person—including detoxification support—that they started to feel well.

What follows is a compilation of my years of research into this area—combining the wisdom of ancient methods such as Ayurvedic medicine with modern science to bring about optimal health and well-being. This book is much more than a one-time detox prescription; it's an opportunity to transform your life with a comprehensive plan for cleaning things up on biological, personal, and social levels. Taking any one of the "Action Steps" in this plan will lead you down the path to a healthier life, and the more steps you take, the more benefit you'll receive.

In Part 1, "Awareness," we look at the scope of the problem of environmental toxins and how they impact our health. We examine why this is such an important issue for us today, where toxins come from, and where they show up in our lives. Through patient examples, you'll see the many ways environmental toxins can gum up our systems and cause health problems that can improve when we apply detoxification and rejuvenation techniques.

In Part 2, "Assessment," we explore what toxins are and how they get into our bodies. You'll assess your level of exposure to toxins from physical, chemical, and mental and emotional sources. Then we'll delve into how our body detoxifies naturally, how some individuals can have impairments in this process, and introduce some basic steps to improve our ability to detoxify. We also go into laboratory testing—what's available, what does it show, and is it necessary?

Part 3, "Action," focuses on specific areas in our lives where we may be exposed to toxins and offers practical solutions to reduce or eliminate those exposures. This section is divided into five major areas, providing a complete approach to healthy living that keeps us resilient to toxic exposures and allows us to thrive.

- First, we shine a light on what we eat. Efforts in this realm can have the largest effect on our health, and this is an area over which we can quickly have some control. We'll identify potential toxins in our foods that should be avoided, as well as foods we can eat to help our detoxification systems work more effectively and keep us healthy.

- The next area we explore is what we put on our bodies, which ultimately ends up *in* our bodies due to our skin's ability to absorb substances. We'll take a detailed look at sources of exposure in our personal care products and clothing and highlight healthy alternatives and fixes.

- We'll then examine the places where we live, work, and play and learn how to look for and deal with common toxins in your home, garage, yard, and workplace.

- Beyond our physical environment, we'll also tackle our mental environment by improving our ability to handle mental and emotional toxicity. This is an area that is often overlooked in detox programs, but can be a key to mental as well as physical wellness.

- And finally, we'll look beyond ourselves to consider what we can do on a social level to control toxic pollutants and reduce their impact on us and the planet.

And so, for the sake of our children, our planet, and ourselves, I offer you practical advice and actions that you can take to tame your toxins and live a healthier and more sustainable, resilient life. Along with my patients, I have cleaned up my diet, my body, my home, and my life in search of optimal health and well-being. By following this plan, you too can get to the root of what's ailing you, creating a better you as well as a better world.

Part 1.
Awareness

Chapter 1.
Our Toxic Burden

It's time to come to terms with the fact that we are all toxic. This may strike you as surprising, but recent studies show this is true. Not only have the amount of man-made chemicals and other pollutants released into the environment dramatically increased over the last century, but the numbers and levels of these toxins accumulating in our bodies have also increased. Hundreds of man-made chemicals are now found in babies at birth,[1] and we then face a lifetime of cumulative exposure from a myriad of sources (natural and unnatural) that add to our total toxic load. Our natural detoxification systems are being pushed to the limit—by the sheer amount of toxins we are exposed to, by the lack of supporting nutrients due to our modern diets, and by genetic differences that can alter our ability to handle toxins—and the result is a toxic buildup! When these toxins are not adequately cleared, our body systems become affected, we are apt to feel fatigued, and we can become ill.

Illnesses Linked to the Environment
Cancer
Autoimmune illness
Asthma

---

1 All women should detoxify regularly prior to conception as many of our accumulated toxins are able to pass to the fetus.

Chronic Fatigue
Birth Defects
Miscarriage
Infertility
Neurologic problems
ADHD
Thyroid disorders
Premature or abnormal sexual development
Headaches
Behavioral disorders
Diabetes
Overweight/Obesity

What is a Toxin?

A toxin is a substance that harms the human body leading to death, disease, or injury. Many can be man-made (synthetic), such as pesticides and industrial chemicals. (The proper term for synthetic toxins is "toxicants," but I will refer to all harmful substances as "toxins" throughout this book for simplicity of understanding.) Toxins also occur in nature, such as heavy metals like lead and arsenic, naturally-occurring gases, infectious agents, and mycotoxins, which are volatile organic compounds (VOCs) released by certain types of mold. Some toxic substances may also physically interfere with the body, such as electromagnetic fields (EMFs) and particulate matter (e.g., soot and smog). And although not commonly acknowledged in the scientific literature, most of us are familiar with toxic emotions, thoughts, and relationships.

Speaking more broadly then, a toxin is anything that is incompatible with a healthy life. Taking this holistic view, most toxins don't necessarily have a skull-and-crossbones label or a neatly placed hazard symbol on them to warn us of their danger. Nevertheless, you can see that toxicity is lurking in our environment at all times, and how we handle it is key to our health and well-being.

Why are Toxins a Problem Now?

In today's world, we are exposed to a constant a barrage of toxins that our bodies are struggling to handle. Not only do we have a background level of naturally occurring toxins, but our environment has changed, bringing about new challenges. As an example, since World War II (WWII) the number of synthetic chemicals in our world has increased dramatically to more than 84,000 unique types in use today. These are designed to be useful, but what do we really know about them? Alarmingly, very few of these chemicals have ever been tested for safety, and none have been tested in the mixture of "chemical soup" that we are exposed to daily, which may create additive or synergistic effects. Many of the chemicals in current use, such as the pesticides, herbicides, and fungicides used in agriculture, were repurposed from their original use as chemical weapons in WWII. Many others, including plastics and much of our cosmetic and personal care products, are derived from petroleum, a by-product of our fossil fuel-based society.

With our prosperous post-WWII economy and a society that demanded convenience and saving time, chemicals designed to help us live easier became so pervasive that 62,000 synthetic chemicals were already on the market and unregulated when the Toxic Substances Control Act (TSCA) was set forth by the US government in 1976. This federal law was specifically designed to allow the Environmental Protection Agency (EPA) to regulate chemicals before they entered into commerce. But all 62,000 of the chemicals on the market before the law took effect were grandfathered in and were assumed safe until proven otherwise by the EPA. An uphill battle from the start, only about 200 of these chemicals have been tested and only six have been partially regulated so far. Meanwhile, 20,000 more chemicals have been allowed into the market without being fully assessed for toxic impact on human health and the environment. Unfortunately, in most cases, the onus is on the consumer to prove harm rather than for the manufacturers to prove safety. And these aren't just chemicals used in a lab: These are in our foods, personal care and cleaning products, food and beverage containers, fabrics, furniture, electronics, toys and other children's products, building materials, and car interiors. We are swimming in a noxious sea of chemical soup, and it is fair to say that we know little of the health effects of exposure. Although a reform of TSCA was signed into law in 2016, the pace of change will be slow due to the backlog of chemicals to be evaluated and the lack of resources to do so.

What we do know is that not only are these chemicals pervasive in the environment, with DDT (a pesticide banned from use by the United States in the 1970s) being found even in the polar ice cores, but these chemicals can also be found in the bodies of every person on the planet. They are everywhere on Earth and are now found in every living thing. We know this because of biomonitoring studies conducted in the United States and around the world. For example, the National Human Adipose Tissue Survey (NHATS), conducted each year from 1970 to 1989, was established by the EPA to collect and analyze human fat tissue specimens from surgical samples and cadavers for the presence of toxic chemicals. They looked across age groups throughout the whole country, testing for polychlorinated biphenyls (PCBs), pesticides, phthalates, and other synthetic chemicals. By the 1980s, numerous toxins such as dioxin (which is carcinogenic, causes reproductive and developmental problems, damages the immune system, and interferes with hormones) and multiple solvents (which can affect the nervous and immune systems) were found in 100 percent of all human fat samples. Every single person sampled contained multiple toxins!

What's even more alarming is that we don't have to be exposed over a long time period of time to have these toxins in us. A study by the Environmental Working Group (EWG) in 2005 showed that before even taking their first breath of life, newborn babies have an average of 200 toxins in their umbilical cord blood. A total of 287 chemicals with known harmful effects were detected in these babies, including 217 neurotoxins and 180 carcinogens such as mercury, lead, PCBs, bisphenol A (BPA), phthalates, plasticizers, and flame retardants. As we are exposed to more toxins in our environment throughout life, our burden increases. Scientists estimate that everyone alive today carries within her or his body at least 700 toxic contaminants.

A Rise in Environmental Illnesses

Research has shown that hundreds of cancer-causing, brain-damaging, and hormone-changing chemicals are found in us at the start of life, and the number goes up as you age. We are also exposed to physical stressors such as man-made electro-magnetic fields that have increased steadily in the last century. Our eating patterns have changed, and we have developed more sedentary lifestyles with high emotional stress. All of these factors can have significant impact on our health and well-being. Therefore, it's no wonder that we're seeing epidemics of diseases such as cancer, obesity, dementia, attention deficit disorder, autism, thyroid disease, and autoimmune disorders, even with all of our medical and scientific advancements. The United States has higher health care costs than any other country and access to the most premier minds and technologies; however, we rank at the bottom of the eleven most industrialized nations on multiple health outcomes. And as a nation we are getting sicker and sicker. We are going beyond our tipping point and becoming tox-sick!

The writing has been on the wall since Rachel Carson published her eye-opening book *Silent Spring* in 1962, calling attention to the impact that technological progress was having on the natural world. These consequences have further progressed, and an example is the continuing rise in cancer cases. At the time of the release of Carson's book, cancer affected one in four people in the United States. Despite the efforts of the "War on Cancer," launched by President Nixon in 1971 to increase research and development of treatments as well as other privately funded efforts, our rates of cancer have increased in the last fifty years to now affect one in two men and one in three women. In other words, 50 percent of men and 33 percent of women in the United States will have cancer within their lifetimes. We do have better and earlier diagnosis, more and better treatments and therapies, and increased survival rates. However, we also have more risk than ever of having cancer in our lifetime. And we are not alone in this: the statistics are increasing across the globe with cancer cases expected to surge 57 percent worldwide in the next twenty years according to the World Health Organization's 2014 World Cancer Report.

The admirable goal of many is to find a cure for cancer and other diseases, but what are we doing to prevent these illnesses in the first place? While environmental influences may not be the sole cause for these diseases, every one of these conditions has an environmental component that should be addressed to reduce toxic effects on our body's basic functioning, including inflammation and genetic changes. If we do, we will wage a much more effective war against these illnesses and could potentially see a decrease in morbidity and mortality rates similar to the steady fall of new cases of lung cancer that came about after the Surgeon General finally called attention to the health hazards of cigarettes in 1964 and urged people not to smoke. It is time to fully acknowledge that our health is intricately connected to our environment and address this root cause of illness.

How Are We Exposed?

At the time of this writing, news headlines point to some major environmental contaminations threatening public health. For example, after a change in water sourcing, Flint, Michigan, became the poster child for devastating lead contamination of tap water that resulted in an epidemic of lead-poisoned children and a potential link to decreased fertility rates and increased fetal death rates. Subsequently, a report by the Natural Resources Defense Council (NRDC) found that the extent of lead contamination of drinking water is much more widespread, with more than eighteen million Americans getting their drinking water from systems with lead contamination. In other news, residents were evacuated from the San Fernando Valley area in California in 2016 after a massive toxic methane gas leak from an underground storage facility was discovered. The leak persisted for months and created symptoms such as nausea, vomiting, headaches, and respiratory problems and contributed to the worst man-made greenhouse gas leak in US history.

We don't have to live in a contamination zone, work in a factory, live near a smokestack or a toxic waste dump, or work on an agricultural farm to be exposed to environmental pollutants, however. We accumulate toxins in our typical everyday lives. We are exposed through the food we eat, the water we drink, what we put on our skin, and the air we breathe. The way we eat has changed substantially in the last century, and this is one of the biggest areas that we can control. Our convenience-based society is heavily reliant on highly processed, cheap, low-quality foods. Current government food labeling requirements can lead to confusion about what is "natural" and "healthy," as well as what exact ingredients and nutrients are in the food. Our conventional crops are grown on tainted, low-nutrient soils, and are sprayed with billions of pounds of toxic pesticides, herbicides, and fungicides. Crops that are heavily subsidized by the US government, such as corn, wheat, and soybeans, have become ubiquitous ingredients in our processed and packaged foods—ingredients to which an increasing number of people have become sensitive. Processed, nutrient-poor foods are cheap and readily available while nutrient-dense whole foods are not, contributing to our epidemics of obesity, diabetes, and inflammatory conditions, including cardiovascular disease and cancer. This is particularly evident in "food deserts"—low-income areas where there are fewer grocery stores and supermarkets, making it challenging to access healthy, affordable food. As a society, we have gone astray from eating in a way that supports our survival and our health.

The water we consume is also a potential route of exposure to toxins. About 70 percent of the human body and 70 percent of our planet is water, however, only 0.007 percent of Earth's water is accessible and usable for people. Much of our water is polluted—even what comes out of the tap or from a bottle. And many industrial and farming practices have the potential to further contaminate our limited resources. Lead, chromium-6, microplastics, pharmaceuticals, and flame retardants are just some of the chemicals which are contaminating millions of Americans' tap water.

Our skin is our largest organ and another point of interaction with our environment. What we put on our skin is absorbed and taken into our bodies. Therefore, it is important to examine our personal care products, such as cosmetics, body creams and lotions, deodorants, shampoos, and perfumes, as they can be a source of exposure. Unfortunately, current regulations do not protect the consumer from potentially harmful ingredients, and we can be exposed to hundreds of chemicals per day just through these products.

Our respiratory tract is another major interface with our environment. We inhale and exhale to breathe between 17,000 to 30,000 times per day, taking in oxygen from the air and removing carbon dioxide and other gases from our bodies. But what else is in the air that we breathe? We may not be aware of invisible toxic exposures such as chlorinated by-products from the steam in our showers, particulate matter from outside air, and volatile organic compounds from chemicals in our home and office.

Other invisible toxins include electromagnetic fields as well as mental and emotional toxins. Paying attention to our exposure to these sources of environmental toxicity can drastically reduce the potential harms of these ubiquitous pollutants. In the following sections, you'll learn how to identify where you may be affected by toxins in your life and find steps you can take to decrease their harmful effects.

What Can We Do About It?

It's easy to become disheartened and overwhelmed when we feel like we have to protect ourselves from 84,000 synthetic chemicals and more. This information isn't meant to cause anxiety, but rather to give us a solid understanding of what our bodies are up against in this day and age. When we are aware, we can choose to reduce exposures to these hazardous situations and optimize our bodies' abilities to handle the toxins that we cannot avoid. By doing this, we become resilient. Sustainable local, national, and global policies would help to reduce widespread pollutants, but there are steps that we can take individually to protect our own microenvironments. Although we cannot immediately solve the problem of global environmental pollution, we can control what we eat, what products we use, the way we breathe, and how well we eliminate toxins from our bodies. We are built to adapt and be able to respond to stresses and different situations. We just need to support our changing needs. As you will see in the next chapter, sometimes shifting even one thing can make a significant impact on our health and well-being. An added bonus to making these healthy lifestyle choices is that we are also contributing to environmentally-friendly and sustainable practices.

"The trees are our lungs, the rivers our circulation, the air our breath, and the earth our body."– Deepak Chopra

Chapter 2. Environmental Toxicity: A Missing Link to Health

The current modern medical approach often focuses on disease management rather than addressing the root cause of illness to restore health. Each major health issue is looked upon as a separate problem that is dealt with in isolation by a specific diagnosis-based treatment, and, particularly for patients with multiple chronic health issues, this can often miss the bigger picture. For example, you may see your cardiologist for your heart disease, your endocrinologist for your diabetes, your rheumatologist for your arthritis, your gastroenterologist for your digestive issues, and your dermatologist for your skin condition—all of them giving you treatments in each of their individual areas, but with none looking at the core underlying problems that set you up for all of these different problems. Many of my patients thought they were doing the right things to improve their health, but the advice they were following wasn't tailored to their individual needs and often neglected toxicity that was hindering the body's ability to heal itself and come back into balance. As you'll see in the following patient examples, finding and addressing the missing links can be the key to healing, particularly with chronic and "unexplained" health problems.

Sara: Doing All the Right Things and Still Not Losing Weight

Sara, a 27-year-old event planner, came to me in tears because she could not lose any of her extra forty pounds despite diet after diet. "I know people think that I am lying or sneaking food, but I swear to you I am not," she pleaded. For the last six months, she had made another valiant effort, exercising vigorously for sixty minutes every day and consuming fewer calories with three vegetarian meals and two small snacks. She drank water and nothing else, giving up coffee and alcohol. But the weight did not budge, and she was seriously frustrated. It seemed the old equation of "calories in and calories out" did not apply to her at all. As we went through her diet in detail, it became apparent that since becoming vegetarian five years prior, she had drastically increased her intake of soy. She had a soy-based protein smoothie in the morning, ate tofu and other soy-based products as meat and dairy substitutes, and grazed on edamame (soy) beans as a healthy snack. Despite doing everything "right," I suspected that her body was reacting to the soy and possibly also causing her thyroid—the body's metabolic regulator—to not function right. Even before the blood tests came back to confirm my suspicions, by going off of soy completely, she started to lose weight and feel better. Soy itself is not necessarily bad, but it was definitely not the right choice for Sara. She is not unlike many of my patients who have held onto excess weight, or suffered from a variety of symptoms from rashes to brain fog, simply because they were eating foods that were not right for their body. When you become sensitive to a food, you may not have a typical allergic-type reaction like rashes, swelling, or digestive upset, and it may not show up on allergy tests. And even though a food may be regarded as "healthy," to some people it can be another source of toxicity: no one diet is good for all people. In Chapter 5, we will look at ways to optimize and individualize our diets so that we can get the most nutrient value and least-toxic load from our foods. This is a stable foundation for healthy living. Focusing on diet alone, however, misses out on an opportunity to fully optimize our health and well-being. For many, like the patient in the next example, we have to look further to discover what's blocking the path to health.

Christopher: A Body Overwhelmed

Christopher was a 32-year-old successful salesman who had put on thirty-five pounds since college. Friendly and gregarious, he enjoyed celebrating his successes with friends by dining on gourmet meals and craft beer. Because he focused so much on his work, he became more sedentary and went to the gym infrequently. When a friend at work lost weight by doing the Master Cleanse fast, he was inspired and followed suit. To follow the Master Cleanse regimen (also known as the Lemonade Diet), he started the morning with a saltwater "flush," drank six to ten glasses of a concoction of maple syrup, lemon juice, cayenne, and water throughout the day, and consumed nothing else. The pounds started to melt off, but after about a week, he developed an itchy rash that soon spread over his entire body. After trying over-the-counter creams to no avail, he went to his primary care doctor who checked his labs (his complete blood count and metabolic panel were normal) and gave him a prescription for a topical steroid cream and an oral antihistamine. When those didn't work, he was given even stronger prescriptions, but nothing helped and the rash continued. After a few weeks of this, he wound up in my office still itching like crazy, despite having finished the Master Cleanse weeks prior.

As I listened to his full story, I realized that as he had lost the weight, he had likely liberated stored toxins from his dissolving reserves of fat, releasing them into his bloodstream and causing the rash. With little protein, calories, or nutrients consumed while on the cleanse, his body was overwhelmed and unable to handle his toxic load. A blood test revealed the likely culprit—he had severely elevated levels of pesticides commonly used on conventional produce in his body. By assisting his body to fully eliminate these toxins instead of allowing them to continue to circulate, he eventually got relief.

Other patients have had effects worse than an itchy rash, such as neurological symptoms, when releasing a large amount of toxins into their bloodstream during rapid weight-loss. So let this be a warning: before any drastic weight-loss or fat-burning program is begun, the toxic load in the body must be reduced *first*. In fact, cleaning up the body's toxic load may be a secret to weight loss. Recent studies indicate that some of these chemicals commonly found in our environment may be what scientists are now calling obesogens—chemicals that the body cannot effectively handle and that potentially affect the hormonal and other systems. These chemicals cause the body to hold on to weight to dilute the toxic effects, and as long as these toxins are in our bodies, the tendency is to gain and hold on to excess weight. This may be one reason why it can be so hard to lose weight or feel better even though we're seemingly doing all of the "right" things.

While food is the biggest potential source of exposure on a daily basis, there are many ways that toxins can impact us. Some may be readily evident and some may take more effort to discover. Sometimes patients need to dig deep to find out what toxic burden has been tipping them over the edge to ill health.

Celine: The Hidden Toxin

A lot of my patients come to me already on what would be considered a "healthy" regimen—eating a mostly plant-based diet, exercising, managing their stress, taking nutritional supplements, etc.—and yet still feel sick and miserable. Take Celine, a 45-year-old mom from the Los Angeles area who gave up her yoga and Pilates studio due to pain and fatigue from an auto-immune nerve disease causing a burning pain in her feet that had started eight years before she consulted me. She had been treated with the very best that conventional medicine could offer, ultimately getting a procedure called plasmapheresis (where blood is removed, filtered, and replaced in the body) every two weeks. Medications including steroids, intravenous immunoglobulins, and chemotherapy had made her feel worse. Despite her illness and debilitating symptoms, she worked hard to improve her health. She did Pilates three times a week, ate a mostly-vegetarian and organic diet, and got eight hours of sleep a night. I had seen many cases like hers that had turned around after a week of cleansing and rejuvenating treatments with us at the Chopra Center and then continuing the lifestyle practices and recommendations at home, so I was hopeful that we could help.

And we did help, a little. Her pain decreased, but it was still there and she was still fatigued. It was time to dig deeper. Looking further into her case, I discovered that she had several food sensitivities and digestive issues that we addressed, and she began to feel stronger after several months. Then, she overdid it at a three-day conference and ended up needing to spend most of her days in bed, and her pain worsened again. Because of financial limitations, she had not yet completed a functional nutritional evaluation or toxicity screen. I explained that it was imperative at this point, and she agreed to do some of the testing. The results revealed that she did have several nutrient deficiencies as well as a genetic tendency that reduced her ability to clear toxins. More importantly, her blood styrene levels were off the charts. Styrene is a petroleum by-product used to make plastics and resins that is considered toxic, mutagenic, and possibly carcinogenic.

After reviewing the possible sources for her exposure (Is it in her drinking water? Does she use Styrofoam products?), we eventually honed in on her breast implants as a possible source of her toxin overload. Several studies have suggested a link between breast implants and autoimmune illnesses, and although she was reluctant to remove the implants, we had not identified any other plausible explanation. When she finally did have the implants removed, she noted immediately after surgery that the burning pain in her feet was gone for the first time in years. She continues to work on her health, balancing her body's challenged detoxification system with a life in the polluted Los Angeles basin. Since she cannot move from the area at this time, she does what she can to mitigate environmental effects and keep her detoxification system working as well as it possibly can by following many of the steps outlined in this book.

In some cases, we cannot adequately control a toxic situation with simple fixes and must take more drastic measures like moving out of or fixing an entire home, such as what happened to Erin Brockovich (not my patient) and several of my patients who lived in homes with toxic mold. In a strange twist of fate, Brockovich, who helped trace illnesses in a small California town to groundwater contaminated by Pacific Gas and Electric, used bonus money she earned from that case to purchase a toxic home. For more than a year, she and her family suffered from flu-like symptoms caused by mold toxins from the black mold *Stachybotrys*. Removing the mold requires highly trained professionals and a lot of protection to prevent further contamination. The estimated expense to fix Brockovich's million-dollar home was about $600,000!

Brenda: Mold, the Toxin That Keeps on Giving

Brenda, a 54-year-old professional, consulted me for help with chronic fatigue syndrome that developed after her apartment flooded and became moldy. Even after moving, she continued to suffer despite improving her nutrition, exercising, and using techniques to deal with mental stress. Why was she still suffering? Her brother lived in a moldy house and each time she visited, she became re-exposed to mold toxins. Even after she stopped going to his house, she continued to be re-exposed every time she came into contact with him or a relative who had visited with him because their clothes and belongings also became infested with toxic mold. Then she discovered she had mold in her new home and had it remediated at a considerable cost, but she still was dealing with fatigue after the repairs.

It turned out that the replacement flooring in her home was off-gassing chemicals that continued to make her sick because she had become sensitized. She had to keep circling back to find the sources of toxic exposure and addressing each one. She kept at it, examining her environment and making changes as needed, and her health is continuing to improve. Despite her sensitivity to the mold in her brother's home, her brother appeared fine. Why? Genetic testing revealed that she was predisposed to not be able to handle toxins well, and her brother probably didn't have this genetic predisposition. To overcome this obstacle, she requires a solid diet, additional nutritional supplementation, and regular detoxification assistance through prescribed cleanses. She is also diligent about avoiding exposures to environmental toxins.

Through my work with these and other wonderful, dedicated patients, I discovered the next evolution of providing truly holistic healthcare. Beyond diets and physical activity, beyond mental and emotional well-being, beyond supplements and detoxes, we need to focus on environmental cleansing—both inside and out—to fully address the root cause of illness and optimize the body's ability to heal. To enjoy the fruit of good health, we truly need to nourish the root and set a better foundation by reducing our total toxic load. For most of my patients, it was not just one thing that affected their health, but rather the sum total of all of their accumulated toxic exposures that tipped them over an invisible line between illness and wellness. Combining my knowledge of Ayurvedic, Functional, and Environmental Medicine, I recognized that every layer needs to be optimized—from what we can see at the concrete level of the body to more subtle levels of the spirit. Although some people require specific focused interventions, there are many simple things that almost anyone can do to shift the needle from more toxic to less toxic. We'll explore how in the rest of this book.

Part 2.

Assessment

Chapter 3.
How Toxic Are You?

Although those who are not particularly sensitive to environmental pollutants may wonder if they are toxic, the question really is *"How* toxic are you?" We are all exposed and have accumulated multiple toxic substances in our bodies, giving us our personal total toxic load. Each of us has an innate ability to detoxify that allows us to handle toxins up to a certain point without noticing any bodily harm or negative health changes. This ability to detox is different in each person and is highly variable. In some cases, the ability to detoxify is impaired, leading to further build-up of toxicity. When our toxic load exceeds our ability to detoxify, our body can be pushed over the tipping point, bringing about symptoms of ill health or disease. The tipping point may result from a single acute exposure, several acute exposures, or a buildup of lower level exposures over a long period of time. Usually, it's not just one thing in isolation that has caused you to feel unwell. For example, it's probably not just that you ate too much tuna and now you have elevated mercury—that is likely just the tip of the iceberg. More realistically, it's the excess tuna, plus the foam mattress that you sleep on, plus the anti-aging miracle cream that you have been slathering on your face daily, combined with foods that are not ideal for your body, that have built up your toxic load. Just doing a quick juice cleanse or lowering one exposure level may get us below a certain threshold, a personal tipping point, but in order to shift the scales back to wellness and achieve optimal functioning and health we need to reduce the total body burden and make sure our detoxification system is working well.

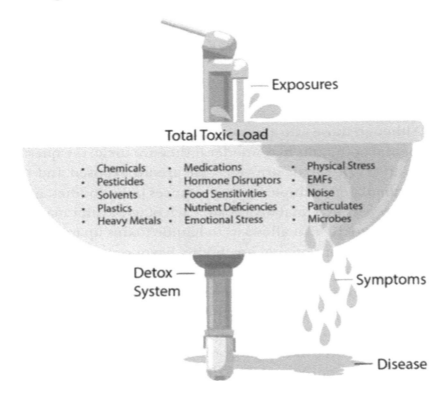

Illustration 1: Our total toxic load is a result of our accumulated toxic exposures and the ability of our detox system to handle the load. Symptoms appear when toxicity accumulates, disrupting functioning of the body system, and can lead to disease if not resolved.

What's contributing to your body burden? Let's take a quick quiz:
- **Do you use personal care products like cosmetics, deodorant, shampoo, lotion, cream, or perfume?**

- **Do you use plastic or Styrofoam food containers or get them with takeout meals?**
- **Do you drink unfiltered tap water or from plastic water bottles?**
- **Do you use store-bought products to clean your home?**
- **Do you wear shoes in your home?**
- **Do you eat animal products or fish?**
- **Do you eat processed foods?**
- **Do you eat nonorganic, conventionally grown produce?**
- **Do you drive or ride in a car, ride a bus, or ride a bike near cars?**
- **Do you work or live in a building that has no openable windows?**
- **Do you sleep on a foam mattress or have furniture cushioned with foam?**
- **Are pesticides or weed killers sprayed in or around your home?**
- **Do you harbor anger, resentment, or hostility?**
- **Do you often feel overwhelmed or anxious?**

If your answer to any of these questions is yes, then chances are that there are some everyday toxic exposures in your life that need to be tamed. Starting at the most fundamental level and then moving outwards in concentric circles, we'll go through possible exposures and what to do about them in the next section.

Canaries in the Coal Mine

For those of us who are chemically sensitive, we can be acutely aware that our toxin load has gone over an invisible threshold and become unmanageable. We are the canaries in the coal mine, the first ones to detect that something in the immediate environment is toxic and threatens to undermine a healthy life.

Some of us can't even walk down the "Household Cleaners" aisle of the supermarket without headaches or nausea. Some become overwhelmed by the smell of car exhaust or other fumes. Some get annoying facial flushing or headaches from drinking a glass of wine, reading a newspaper, or smelling cigarette smoke. Those of us who have these types of reactions may be regarded as highly sensitive, and even perhaps a little crazy, because many others do not detect these noxious substances at the levels that we do.

In reality, we canary-types are the unfortunate harbingers of our planet's environmental doom. According to a National Academy of Sciences report, 15 percent of the population was chemically sensitive in 1981, and a more recent random population study by the California Department of Health Services showed a similar hypersensitivity prevalence of 15.9 percent in Californians surveyed. People may also be affected without realizing that their symptoms are related to toxic exposures, like many of my patients. In the future, public availability of genetic testing may help identify those who have a potential for a reaction as well as the substances to which they may react. For instance, I have a gene that makes me susceptible to mold toxin, and I can have adverse reactions with mold exposure. I don't think it's any coincidence that I can detect whether there's mold or mildew in a room way before almost anyone else can. It's just my body's way of alerting me to a potential threat to my health.

If you are environmentally sensitive, following the steps outlined in this book can help keep your total toxic load controlled and your detox system optimized. Those who are suffering from severe health challenges or who want more clarity on what exposures to focus on may want to seek out an environmental medicine specialist to help identify the possible problems contributing to ill health. The American Academy of Environmental Medicine and the list of those who have completed Dr. Walter Crinnion's Comprehensive Training in

Environmental Medicine are two referral sources for physicians with this type of training (*see* Resources). In addition to a detailed environmental history and clinical exam, these specialists may offer specific laboratory testing that can help guide treatment.

Is There a Test for Toxins?

At this writing, there are many laboratory tests to detect levels of certain toxic substances in our blood, tissue, or urine, although there is no current method to detect our total body burden. And while more than 80,000 chemicals are registered for daily commercial and industrial use, we have tests to check for only about 250 of them. Many of the most common offenders can be measured through standard and specialty lab testing. Standard laboratories can test for heavy metals such as lead, arsenic, and mercury, and the cost of some testing may be covered by insurance. To get an accurate picture, however, it is important to order the right test in the right way and interpret it appropriately. For example, finding elevated heavy metals in a hair sample alone doesn't really tell about heavy metal toxicity or the state of your toxic load. There are many other variables to consider, so I recommend working with an environmental specialist who is trained in this area. Testing for some substances may require specialty laboratories that are often not covered by insurance and can be quite expensive. However, we should seriously consider spending money for certain tests when there is a potential to discover the root cause of illness, particularly if we have tried a number of treatments and continue to feel unwell. Many of my patients choose to invest in their health and get testing done. In some situations, testing is important in determining a course of treatment. For instance, some health practitioners and promoters of natural supplements claim that certain foods, herbs, or nutrients are beneficial for heavy metal chelation (a process of one substance binding with another substance to increase elimination). However, it would take an awfully long time and a boatload of cilantro/chlorella/insert-latest-fad-here to reduce a truly toxic heavy metal load. When lab testing confirms that heavy metals are significantly elevated in the body, a reputable health care provider may prescribe a safe and effective chelating regimen and monitor your progress. Heavy metal poisoning can cause many serious health problems and should be treated by practitioners experienced in this area.

What About Genetic Testing?

Genetic testing involves examining your DNA, the blueprint that carries instructions for your body's structure and functions. Although there are limitations, genetic testing can reveal differences in your genes that may cause illness or disease. For some people, knowing about genetic tendencies regarding the ability to detoxify may be important, but this can also be a costly out-of-pocket expense (although prices have come down in recent years). A few tests may be covered by insurance depending on your health condition and family history, such as BRCA (breast cancer tumor suppressor gene) testing for those with a personal or family history of breast and ovarian cancer or MTHFR (methylenetetrahydrofolate reductase enzyme gene) testing for those with heart disease. Other tests, such as those that evaluate genetic differences in Phase I and Phase II liver enzymes that are used to metabolize toxins (as described in the next chapter) may be an out-of-pocket expense. Knowing if we have problems detoxifying or metabolizing certain substances does not necessarily rubber stamp us for illness. Most of our genes have variable expression, meaning the things that we do and the environment in which we live have the ability to turn these genes on and off. We can utilize this knowledge to be preventative; we can be more aware of and reduce toxic exposures that we are prone to have difficulty with and use foods, nutrients, and other techniques to overcome deficiencies and optimize our body's functioning as much as possible, turning health genes on and disease genes off.

Daryl: Looking Beyond the Standard Risk Factors

A good example of how awareness of genetic tendencies influences the course of treatment is demonstrated with Daryl, a 57-year-old executive who was healthy until a few years prior to his visit when he began to have bouts of chest pain. Over the course of a year, he had been evaluated by a heart specialist, lung specialist, and gastrointestinal specialist, who all found nothing wrong. But he started to have increasing chest pain and shortness of breath when hiking and returned to his general practitioner who ordered a treadmill stress test. During the test, he had chest pain and was sent for immediate cardiac catheterization where they found four blockages in the arteries providing blood flow to his heart. He received an angioplasty to open the clogged arteries and a stent was placed to keep it open. In recovering from these procedures, he unfortunately suffered a heart attack. Attempts to repeat angioplasty procedures to the affected arteries failed, and he ended up needing open heart surgery with a quadruple bypass. Despite having normal cholesterol, normal blood pressure, no family history of heart problems, and a non-smoking, healthy lifestyle, he endured this great trauma to his health and was placed on blood pressure and cholesterol medications that made him feel poorly. He came to me for assistance in living with the diagnosis of heart disease. I was able to give him some additional diet and lifestyle recommendations, but I also wanted to look further into possible hidden contributing factors since he didn't have any of the typical known risk factors that are seen with heart disease. Did he have a certain genetic issue making him prone to atherosclerosis? Did his nutrient and toxin levels contribute to disease onset? Based on lab testing, we discovered that he did have a genetic condition that predisposed him to blood clots, and his vitamin and nutrient levels needed to be optimized to keep his blood vessels healthy. He also had elevated heavy metals (lead, mercury, and cadmium) that are associated with heart disease. To achieve total well-being, all of these areas needed to be addressed. In addition to eating a balanced diet, he took nutritional supplements to address any deficiencies and we monitored his progress with follow-up labs. He also underwent chelation therapy with a qualified professional to bring down his heavy metal levels. Today he continues to do well, enjoying an active lifestyle with no further symptoms.

Regardless of whether or not lab testing is done to evaluate for toxic accumulations, reducing exposures and optimizing our detoxification systems moves us in the right direction. Going back to Illustration 1 of our total toxic body burden, imagine a sink with a water faucet turned on and a clogged drain causing water to overflow onto the floor. Instead of standing in the quagmire, continually mopping the floor in an attempt to mask the end result of overflowing water, we need to turn off the faucet and unclog the drain to get to the root of the problem and achieve a long-term fix. This scenario is akin to possible actions we can take when confronted with health problems. Continually mopping up is comparable to the use of pharmaceuticals for symptom management in many situations. However, rather than just masking or reducing symptoms, we need to fix the faucet by identifying and addressing the contributing factors that led to the health problem, which may include exposure to toxins. Additionally, we can unclog the drain by revving up our detoxification systems so that our bodies are able to properly function and eliminate unwanted and hazardous substances. Even when the cause of an illness hasn't been specifically identified, reducing the total toxic load and optimizing the detoxification system helps to promote health. We'll learn how in the rest of this book.

Figuring Out Your Toxic Body Burden

Shifting your habits and making changes in your everyday environment can drastically reduce your exposure and lower your total body burden. But where do you start? Part 3 of this book is divided into major areas where we accumulate toxicity in our lives, and each area is further broken down into more manageable chunks to focus on. For each area, look at your personal exposures to toxic insults as well as your individual susceptibility to their effects. Then you can choose to take steps to lower your body burden. What you consume as food and beverages is one of the biggest areas to address toxic exposures and also impacts how well your detoxification system is working, so that should be primary. In Chapter 5, you'll learn how to eat well to lay the foundation for good health. The next area to take control of is where your exposure may be the greatest. Perhaps it is what you put on your body. The average American adult uses nine personal care products each day, with 126 unique chemical ingredients—that's quite a cocktail! We explore this area and what to do about it in Chapter 6. You may also have some major exposures in the place where you spend the most time, usually the home, which we tackle in Chapter 7. In particular, the bedroom may need some attention, since most of us spend about one-third of our lives in bed. These chapters provide simple Action Steps to clean up your personal environment and possibly save money as well.

Chapter 4.
Is Your Detox
System Optimized?

How Do Our Bodies Detoxify?

Our bodies are constantly working to excrete intrinsic toxins produced by natural metabolic processes as well as external toxins that we take in from microbes and natural and man-made chemicals in our air, food, water, and surroundings. Our liver, kidneys, skin, lungs, and intestines all play a role in helping us to detoxify. If these systems are not working effectively to clear toxins from the body, we end up with a toxin buildup. Our total toxic load is the result of our toxic input minus our toxic output; so, in addition to reducing our overall exposure to toxins (taking less in), we need to make sure our detoxification systems are working well to mobilize and remove toxins. Our individual abilities to detoxify determine the amount of toxins that we eliminate or store in our bodies at any given time, so follow the Toxin Tamer Tips below to support your detox system.

How Do Toxins Get in Your Body?

Many people are familiar with the phrase "You are what you eat," but we really are the product of *everything* in our environment that we ingest, digest, and metabolize. This includes not only the food and beverages that we consume, but also the air that we breathe and the substances that we absorb through our skin. While we may think of the environment as something "out there" that is apart from our body, in reality, there is no separation. We are interwoven and interconnected with the nature of our surroundings. As evidenced by the 2015 Flint, Michigan, water supply tragedy, the rivers are our blood. The trees, supplying vital oxygen, are our breath. The soil, from which plants obtain nutrients that ultimately go up the food chain, is our body. Because we usually don't usually notice a bad effect immediately from these exposures, it's easy to ignore the slow, steady accumulation of toxins which can ultimately have harmful effects. And the effects can go beyond those of just a single toxic substance, as interactions with other chemicals can create potential additive or synergistic effects, increasing the negative impacts.

Aside from our physical bodies and environments, we're also a product of our mental and emotional environments. In the last twenty years, science has confirmed that our mental state and our thoughts can affect our physiology. Your physical complaints and symptoms are not just all in your head. The fundamental levels of our senses—what we see, hear, feel, smell, and taste—are interpreted by our nervous system. If we interpret these experiences negatively, the corresponding physiological responses can also act as "toxins" and harm our body. Studies have shown that simply looking at disturbing images can impact your immune system in addition to influencing your brain. Even at the most basic level, too much or too little light can affect our health. We are affected by what we hear, from words to music to general noise pollution. We are affected by touch—if we are touched, as well as how we are touched. And one of the most primitive of our senses, the sense of smell, not only triggers memories but also can have a direct effect on our nervous system. Taste informs us about food, creating pleasant or unpleasant feelings and sensations. Together, our senses create an impression of the world we are in and our thoughts further refine our perception. In the same way that our senses inform the brain of what is going on, the brain can inform the body of what is happening—sometimes for our benefit, and sometimes not.

Rupa: The Issues in Her Tissues

Beyond a toxic physical environment, we can also have toxic beliefs, toxic emotions, and toxic relationships. Rupa, a 35-year-old Indian-American mother of two, came to see me for chronic neck pain that had not responded to months of medications and physical therapy. She had X-rays and MRIs of her neck that were all normal. She felt the pain constantly for the last two years and was willing to try some of my new suggestions, such as acupuncture. But during our in-depth consultation, we came to a point where she revealed that her mother-in-law moved in with them two years prior. Since that time, she felt that she had no voice and that her opinion was not respected in her own house. She had not shared this with anyone previously, but as she talked with me and was finally able to express her feelings and concerns, she exclaimed, "Oh my God, my neck pain is gone!" By releasing the toxicity of her emotion, she became free of the pain in her neck. Her case is a valid example of the powerful connection between the mind and the body. All of the experiences and feelings that we have make up how we respond to the world and ultimately impact our physiology.

According to Ayurveda, our experiences in life (food, sensory experiences, and emotions) are metabolized by a digestive fire known as *agni* [pronounced *ahg-nee*]. This digestive fire is responsible not only for processing physical substances from the macroscopic to the microscopic levels, but also for processing our thoughts and emotions. If we have a strong digestive fire, we are able to extract the nutrients from our food and molecules of emotion from our thoughts that allow us to feel vibrant and alive, while releasing substances that we do not need and that do not serve us. This is described as having *ojas* [pronounced *oh-jahss*], a vital essence. If, however, our digestive fire is weak, then it is similar to having wet logs in a fire. Food and experiences are not fully metabolized and toxic residue known as *ama* [pronounced *ah-ma*] accumulates, clogging our system, leading us to feel fatigued, and impairing our body's functions. This accumulation of *ama* can often be the initiation point of illness, the root of disease that is often not addressed by symptom-masking approaches.

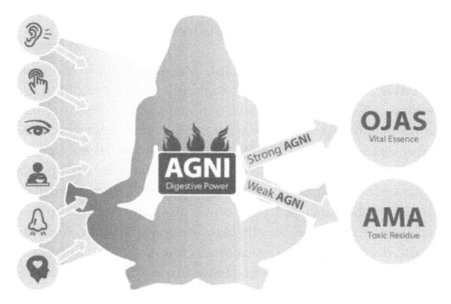

Illustration 2. Agni (digestive capacity) determines if we will metabolize our life experiences into ojas (vital essence) or ama (toxic residue)

Ayurveda: Ancient Healing Wisdom

Ayurveda is a holistic system of medicine from India that is said to have originated about five thousand years ago. It is a science based on principles of nature and utilizes preventive practices as well as specific treatments to bring the mind, body, and spirit back into balance to restore health. Treatments are based on a person's unique constitution, known as *dosha* [pronounced *doh-sha*], and include lifestyle recommendations, herbal remedies, and cleansing practices. Meditation and yoga, sister sciences of Ayurveda, are core practices that facilitate mind-body balance. Ayurveda, meditation, and yoga have become increasingly popular in Western culture, and recent scientific research is validating many of the purported benefits. See the Resources section if you are interested in learning more.

This concept of *agni* explains why some people can make lifestyle choices known to be harmful (such as smoking and eating a diet of highly processed foods) and not appear to have any ill health effects. They are the ones who are blessed with a strong *agni*, and as the old Ayurvedic saying goes, their digestive fire is strong enough to metabolize effectively to "turn poison into nectar." On the other side, however, I have seen many patients who supposedly are doing all of the "right" things—they eat an organic, locally-grown vegetarian diet, meditate daily, do yoga, and are emotionally balanced –but because of their inherently weak *agni*, they cannot fully metabolize all this goodness and end up with residue turning "nectar into poison" and causing dysfunction and disease in their bodies.

Toxin Tamer Tip #1: Digest to be Your Best

The state of our digestive fire can be changed for better or worse. It shifts with time of day, what we consume (including medications and herbs), and lifestyle habits. Many of my patients have unfortunately dampened their *agni* by doing such things as overeating, undereating, eating at the wrong time, eating the wrong food for their needs or the wrong combination of foods, making drastic dietary changes, sleeping excessively or too little, living in extreme climates, having physical stress from illness, injury, or excessive physical activity, and holding onto emotional stress. We all know that these things can make the difference between feeling well and unwell. The good news is that by optimizing what we eat, aligning our lifestyle with the cycles of nature, and utilizing ancient techniques to enhance the body's capacity to heal, we can jump-start our *agni* so that our ability to digest food, experiences, and emotions can lead us down the harmonious path to health rather than the rancid road to disease.

We are more than what we eat; we are what we digest—a sum total of our unique responses to all of our collective experiences—and this is why we must go beyond just cleaning up our diet or doing a quickie detox cleanse. We must address the whole system—mind, body, spirit, and environment—to ensure balance and prevent the accumulation of excess toxicity. You will find specific tools to enhance your physical *agni* in Chapter 5 and your mental and emotional *agni* in Chapter 8.

Toxin Tamer Tip #2: Empty Your "Garbage Can" Daily

What happens when you do not take out your trash on a regular basis? As the garbage can fills up, there is not as much room to handle more, and eventually it overflows, leaving a stinky mess. In a similar way, we also need to take out our bodies' garbage, providing a clear exit path for toxins by moving our bowels (i.e., pooping) regularly. That doesn't mean every fourth day, or even every other day. Regular bowel movements, for most, means at least once per day, if not more. Consider the amount of stuff that we put into the front-end of our gastrointestinal system (i.e., our mouths). If what is coming out at the other end amounts to a few rabbit-poop pellets or a single small bowel movement a day, then you might see why you feel like crap—you are literally full of it! It's not just digested and undigested food stuff that exits from our GI tracts, it is *the* main exit route for toxic compounds. Toxins that are not released in this manner may get reabsorbed from the colon and go right back into the bloodstream, essentially re-toxifying the system. If you tend to be constipated, you are not alone. With our low-fiber, nutrient-poor diet and sedentary lifestyle, millions of Americans have come to rely on laxatives making it a $1-billion-a-year market. Chronic use of stimulant laxatives is not good for you, though, so look to the recommendations in Action Step 9 to literally get yourself going.

Toxin Tamer Tip #3: Let It Flow

The other main exit is via our kidneys through urine. Our kidneys act as a filter, balancing fluids and removing toxins and wastes. Two major things affect kidney function: the amount of liquids we consume, which is why it is so important to drink plenty of clean water, and the pH (acid or alkaline levels) of your urine. In general, the more alkaline the urine, the more toxins are released, while the more acidic the urine, the more toxins are recycled and taken back up into our system. A main way we can decrease acidity and increase alkalinity is by focusing on the foods and beverages that we consume, such as increasing intake of dark leafy greens, which help to create a more alkaline environment. Certain herbs and nutrients can also play a role. See Action Step 1 for more details on alkalinizing foods that can help this system flow.

Toxin Tamer Tip #4: Love Your Liver

Now that our exits are working well, it's time to rev up our main chemical processor, the liver. Toxin-metabolizing enzymes throughout the body initiate the breakdown of toxins. The small intestines and lungs are particularly adept in this manner. Once the toxins are initially metabolized, the remaining components are then shuttled to the kidneys (water-soluble) or liver (fat-soluble) for further processing.

The first step of the liver's detoxification process is called Phase I. During this process, the substance is modified to make it more water-soluble via the cytochrome P450 (CYP450) enzyme system. Currently there are fifty-seven different CYP450 genes known, and these help us metabolize substances such as combustion by-products from charbroiled meats and exhaust fumes, estrogen, nitrosamines, and nicotine, alcohol, and more than 70 percent of all prescription drugs and steroid hormones. Certain nutrients are necessary for this enzyme system to handle these substances properly and include the B vitamins, vitamin C, vitamin E, glutathione, selenium, magnesium, amino acids, carotenes, and flavonoids. We can't even begin to handle our toxic load without these nutrients.

In some cases, Phase I processing makes a substance more active or reactive. For instance, this is the mechanism by which some pharmaceutical drugs convert to their therapeutically active component. This is also the process that turns alcohol to an aldehyde, giving us the unpleasant experience of a hangover. Some substances are turned into cancer-causing compounds or free radicals which can damage tissues, so our bodies need to move them on to Phase II to get them to out of the system.

In Phase II, another molecule is added to make the substance more water-soluble so that it's readily cleared via the kidneys or the bowel, a process called conjugation. Several enzyme systems are responsible for this process (COMT, NAT, GST, SOD, and others), and this phase is crucial for metabolizing neurotransmitters, estrogen, and environmental toxins such as tobacco smoke, exhaust fumes, solvents, herbicides, fungicides, lipid peroxides, and heavy metals. Certain amino acids that we get from protein-rich foods are key co-factors in this step, including N-acetylcysteine (NAC), taurine, glutamine, glycine, cysteine, and methionine. Further details on foods, nutrients, and herbs to help support your liver function are found in Action Step 10.

Phase III is the transport and elimination phase where the toxins that have been made water-soluble are now removed from the cells and from the body. Phase III transporters are present in many tissues, including the liver, kidneys, intestines, and brain, and require energy to pump toxins through the cell membrane and out of the cell. Transporters move the substances created in Phase II out of cells and into the bile and intestines for elimination. In the kidneys, toxins are removed from the blood for urinary excretion. Sweating also helps to remove toxins through the skin. A whole-foods, high-fiber diet rich in deeply pigmented vegetables and fruits is important to support Phase III elimination processes. In addition, microbial balance plays a role as dysbiosis (microbial imbalance) may contribute to deconjugation, essentially reversing what was done in Phase II and allowing the toxins to recirculate back to the liver (enterohepatic recirculation). Elevations in one of the enzymes responsible for deconjugation—beta-glucuronidase—is associated with an increased risk for various cancers including breast, prostate, and colon cancer. Maintaining functioning of this phase is key. When Phase III is impaired, a negative feedback loop results in down-regulation of Phase II enzymes, which can result in buildup of reactive Phase I metabolites which can then further impair detoxification and cause damage.

Toxin Tamer Tip #5: Free Your Mind

All of the detox plans I have seen give advice about diet, and some of them also let you know about toxic products you may be exposed to, but very few address an invisible source of toxicity that can have just as big an impact: your mind. Many of us don't understand our mind's role in creating our experience of life, our emotions, and even our physical health. Instead of steering the ship to create health, we may let our minds run wild, worrying about and projecting toward the future or replaying the past by rehashing mistakes and stewing in grievances and resentments. But by exercising our free will, we can release the past, break free from conditioned responses, accept the present as it is, and be open to the future. If we commit to understanding our roles in creating our own experiences of life, we have an opportunity to manifest different results by making conscious choices.

Bill: Freeing the Mind to Heal the Body

Take the example of Bill, a 35-year-old who came to me for help with severe anxiety, panic disorder, and insomnia. He had served in the US military and was deployed to Iraq and Afghanistan multiple times where he was exposed to several traumatic events that were the cause of Post-Traumatic Stress Disorder (PTSD). He described being on constant alert and reliving events over and over again. He tried to control his feelings and also bottled up anger and resentment, releasing it all to his wife in explosive outbursts that were affecting their marriage. Beyond his mental health concerns, he had also developed high blood pressure, had gained weight, and had pain in both knees. He had been on multiple medications for several years but was not noticing much improvement and knew that something needed to change.

Recognizing that his thoughts were keeping him stuck and possibly contributing to his health decline, Bill decided to take part in the Chopra Center's Healing the Heart weekend program, during which he was guided through an emotional release process designed by Dr. David Simon. Freeing himself from the mental and emotional toxicity that he had been carrying opened him up to the possibility of healing. He began to really take care of himself by meditating twice a day and working on his emotional health and his relationship with his wife. He also started incorporating Ayurvedic principles to live more in balance—eating better, exercising, and improving his bedtime routine. While he did notice a shift in his mental outlook immediately following the weekend program, the true transformation occurred after he diligently implemented these health practices for several months: he noted a lightness of spirit as well as of his body, he lost fifteen pounds, eliminated his knee pain, and reduced his blood pressure medication. He shifted not only his mental outlook, but his entire body.

Are You Ready to Tame Your Toxins and Reclaim Your Health?

In order to fully tame our toxins, we need to mindfully address all of the areas in which we may be exposed with a **complete** plan to detoxify all the layers of life—from the physical body and environment to mental consciousness. Otherwise, we'll perpetually fill up with poisons despite our best efforts to remove them. Unfortunately, we can't trust that all of the products we buy are safe, so we need to read labels and ask questions: Where did this food come from? How was it raised? What are the ingredients in my shampoo, lipstick, and sunscreen? What materials are in my mattress? What's in my water? In Part 3, we take a look at lurking hazards and learn how to take control of the things that we can and let go of the things that we cannot, addressing physical, mental, emotional, and societal toxicity in order to achieve total well-being.

In the next sections, you will find **fifty-two specific Action Steps** designed to address every layer of toxicity in your life and support these general toxin tamer tips:

Toxin Tamer #1: Digest to Be Your Best
Toxin Tamer #2: Take Out Your "Garbage" Daily
Toxin Tamer #3: Let It Flow
Toxin Tamer #4: Love Your Liver
Toxin Tamer #5: Free Your Mind

Taking any Action Step or all of them moves us towards reduced toxicity and increased health. Whether you focus on one Action Step each week or choose to go at your own pace, you will:

- **Optimize your diet to maximize detoxification and digestion and minimize your toxic exposure from foods.**
- **Ditch the toxic products in your home and garden, replacing them with healthy and affordable alternatives.**
- **Reclaim control of your physical and mental environment.**
- **Move towards a lifestyle that creates a healthier you and a healthier planet.**

Join me on the journey to wellness with a complete plan to be *resilient* and thrive.

Part 3.

Action: 52 Steps to Tame Toxins and Reclaim Your Health

Chapter 5.
What Goes In: Food

"Let food be thy medicine and medicine be thy food."
                                              - Hippocrates

Are you confused about what to eat? If so, you are not alone. In the last few years, many long-standing dietary recommendations have been upended, leaving people puzzled about what to do. Cholesterol and fat are no longer public enemy number one, and whole grains, which for the last thirty years have been the stable base of our food pyramid, are now thought of in some circles as poison to our system. Two-thirds of our country is overweight and nearly 10 percent have diabetes, and that number is expected to reach nearly a third of the population by 2050. Time and again, research has shown that what we eat can make an impact on weight, diabetes, and heart disease as well as other health challenges such as cancer, arthritis, and other inflammatory diseases. If we know food is vital to our well-being, why don't we know what to eat?

You don't see animals in the wild wondering what they should eat. They know what food is: it is vitality, it is life. Food is energy to sustain us, in the form of calories from protein, fat, and carbohydrates, and it is information that interacts with the environment; the message is conveyed by the nutrients and phytochemicals (plant-based natural chemicals) to our cells and even to our genome. When we choose the highest quality energy and information for our needs—which we especially get from whole, real foods—our systems work optimally and we move towards balance, health, and vitality.

Cleaning up the foods that we eat is potentially the most effective way we can make an impact on our health. As more people become aware of what foods are beneficial as well as what substances in foods can potentially cause harm, it has become easier for us to find and make healthy choices. However, we do have to pay attention, especially if we're eating out. Follow the basic food rules outlined in this book, and you will not only tame toxins, but also fight disease, achieve a healthy weight, and minimize the effects of aging. The old Ayurvedic saying goes, "When diet is wrong, medicine is of no use. When diet is correct, medicine is of no need." While medications may be necessary to treat some disease conditions, most of my patients improved their health and many were able to reduce or eliminate the need for medications by shifting their dietary and lifestyle habits.

1. Eat a Rainbow

There's no denying that eating a variety of colorful fresh vegetables and fruits is beneficial for your health. Each natural color represents a group of nutrients and phytochemicals that optimizes our bodies' functioning. Aim to eat at least three different colors from natural food sources per day, if not more. When possible, choose organic produce (see Action Step 2). To get the most bang for your buck, make sure to incorporate these colorful detox superfoods as a regular part of your diet.

- **Berries** – Low in sugar and high in fiber, these tasty morsels are high in phytonutrients and antioxidants. Blackberries, blueberries, raspberries, red currants, and strawberries all pack a flavorful nutrient punch.

Antioxidants protect energy-producing mitochondria and prevent oxidative damage which can alter normal cellular processes. Most of the changes we associate with aging are a result of oxidative damage, and all environmental toxins cause oxidative damage. Available year-round, frozen berries may have even more beneficial phytonutrients readily available, as freezing releases the nutrients by breaking cell walls.

- **Broccoli and other cruciferous vegetables** – Brussels sprouts, bok choy, cauliflower, kale, collard greens, cabbage, broccoli sprouts: these veggies contain sulfur compounds, which help to support detoxification and reduce the risk of some cancers, and indole-3 carbinol, which helps process estrogen and testosterone in a healthy way.
- **Dark leafy greens** – Spinach, kale, romaine, collard greens, mustard greens, chard, arugula, and leafy lettuces are a great non-dairy source of calcium. These greens help to alkalinize our blood, optimizing our ability to detoxify and reducing inflammation. They are also a great source of folate, carotenoids, vitamin K, and fiber—key nutrients for detoxification and a healthy body.
- **Avocado** – Packed with monounsaturated fat, which is heart healthy and improves cholesterol levels, avocados are also a good source of fiber, glutathione (an antioxidant important to support detoxification by the liver), folate, and potassium.
- **Red, orange, and yellow vegetables** – Tomatoes, peppers, sweet potatoes, carrots, squash, and beets provide antioxidants and other beneficial phytonutrients. Note that some people can be sensitive to nightshade vegetables, which may be included in this class. If you are dealing with inflammation, you may consider a trial eliminating nightshades from your diet. See the Appendix for more details on how to do an elimination diet.

- **Other fruits** – Choose low sugar fruits that are high in fiber such as apples and cantaloupe. Highly pigmented, colorful fruits contain beneficial nutrients, but be mindful not to overload on sugar even if it is from fruit. Some great lower-sugar fruit choices include: papaya, cantaloupe, kiwi, guava, apples, tart cherries, peaches, oranges, and apricots. Citrus fruits such as lemons and limes can add great flavor, help support digestion, and alkalinize the body.

Nightshade Foods

A particular group of substances in these foods, called alkaloids, may cause symptoms such as joint and muscle pain or digestive disturbances in particularly sensitive people. Foods considered to be nightshades include:

- Potatoes
- Tomatoes
- Many species of sweet and hot peppers
- Eggplant
- Ground cherries (all species of genus *Physalis*)
- Tomatillos
- Garden huckleberry
- Tamarillos
- Pepinos
- Naranjillas
- Pimentos (also called pimientos)
- Goji berries
- Paprika
- Cayenne
- Tabasco sauce

Note: Sweet potatoes, yams, black pepper, and white pepper are not considered nightshades.

Alkalinize to Remove Toxins

Other fruits and vegetables that are rich in acid-buffering minerals such as calcium, sodium, potassium, and magnesium can also help to alkalinize urine, which assists the body's ability to excrete toxins. Most vegetables and sprouted beans are alkalinizing. This property may be part of the reason why plant-based diets can be so healthy. Include some of these alkalinizing foods as part of your regular diet.

Alkalinizing Fruits	Alkalinizing Vegetables	Alkalinizing Nuts, Seeds, and Grains
Apples	Asparagus	Almonds
Apricots	Beets	Fresh coconut
Bananas	Broccoli	Chestnuts
Berries	Brussels sprouts	Flax seeds
Oranges	Cabbage	Pumpkin seeds
Grapefruit	Celery	Sesame seeds
Lemons	Chard	Sunflower seeds
Cantaloupe	Cauliflower	Chia seeds
Cherries	Collard greens	Amaranth
Figs	Cucumbers	Millet
Grapes	Eggplant	Quinoa
Kiwi	Kale	
Mangoes	Lettuce	
Watermelon	Mustard greens	
Honeydew melon	Onions	
Nectarines	Parsnips	
Pineapples	Peppers	
Pear	Pumpkin	
Tangerines	Turnips	
	Sprouts	
	Sweet potatoes	
	Watercress	

2. Choose Organic

While it may not always be possible, choosing organic food reduces your risk of exposure to harmful pesticides and also supports farming practices that are not as destructive to the environment and wildlife. An environmental medicine colleague of mine described a patient who was making an effort to be healthy by consuming a celery and spinach juice daily that was not organic. After a while, the patient noted increases in panic and noise sensitivity, and upon evaluation by my colleague was found to have toxic levels of organophosphate pesticides up to ten times the upper limit. After two weeks off of the nonorganic juice, many of the levels dropped to the nontoxic range and some in the range just above the upper limit. Best of all, his symptoms resolved.

US pesticide usage totaled over 1.1 billion pounds annually in both 2011 and 2012, and the agricultural sector accounted for nearly 90 percent of the total pesticide usage, impacting our food supply. A US Department of Agriculture (USDA) study found that nearly 70 percent of samples of 48 types of conventionally grown produce were contaminated with pesticide residues, with 178 different pesticides and pesticide breakdown products detected. The pesticides persisted on fruits and vegetables even when they were washed and peeled. The different types of chemicals used have different toxic effects. Organophosphate pesticides (OPs) were originally developed as neurological poisons for chemical warfare in World War I and act as a poison to the nervous systems of insects, plants, and humans. High levels of OPs are associated with increased ADHD, decreased IQ, and dementia. A different class called organochlorine pesticides poison insulin-receptor sites, worsen metabolic syndrome and diabetes, and have other effects on hormonal and immune systems. The herbicide atrazine, found in 94 percent of our water supply, has been linked to birth defects, infertility, and cancer. Combinations of these chemicals with other toxic agents such as arsenic and aluminum can have synergistic effects, making matters worse. The good news is that blood levels of these toxins can decrease quickly after switching to organic foods.

Chlorpyrifos: The Nerve Gas Relative That's on Our Food

Chlorpyrifos is an organophosphate pesticide and, by pounds of active ingredient, is the most widely used conventional insecticide in the United States. It is currently used on a large variety of food crops as well as on non-residential turf and ornamental plants. Aside from food, exposure can come from dust that drifts from treated fields into homes and schools as well as from water contamination. CDC data showed chlorpyrifos-related substances in 93 percent of US residents sampled between 1999 and 2002, and children had particularly high levels of chlorpyrifos—almost double that of adults. Farmworkers and people living in agricultural communities, particularly children, are especially affected by this toxic pesticide.

After increasing scientific evidence that chlorpyrifos might be harmful to human health, the EPA prohibited household use in 2001; however, use in public and for agriculture has continued. With additional research suggesting further toxicity concerns including possible links to neurodevelopmental problems, lung and prostate cancer, and endocrine-disrupting potential, the EPA prioritized its review of chlorpyrifos and in 2015, responding to a petition from the Natural Resources Defense Council and the Pesticide Action Network North America, proposed to ban the use of chlorpyrifos. In November 2016, the EPA released a revised human health risk assessment for chlorpyrifos confirming no safe uses. They found that:

- All food exposures exceed safe levels, with children ages 1 to 2 exposed to levels of chlorpyrifos that are 140 times the level that the EPA deems safe.

- No safe level of chlorpyrifos in drinking water exists.
- Drift from spraying reaches unsafe levels at 300 feet from the field's edge.
- In agricultural areas, unsafe levels are found in the air at schools, homes, and communities.
- All workers who mix and apply chlorpyrifos are exposed to unsafe levels even if using maximum personal protective equipment and engineering controls.
- Unsafe exposures continue more than two weeks after application on average, yet field workers are allowed to re-enter fields within one to five days.

Unfortunately, in March 2017 EPA Administrator Scott Pruitt went against the EPA's own conclusions and reversed the proposed ban, allowing chlorpyrifos to remain on the market without providing any new scientific evidence of safety. This chemical poses harmful risks, and US senators from several states agreed, proposing a bill—S. 1624 The Protect Children, Farmers & Farmworkers from Nerve Agent Pesticides Act—that would ban chlorpyrifos. You can protect yourself and your families by purchasing organic fruits and vegetables. Some of the crops that chlorpyrifos is used on include: apples, lettuce, peaches, sweet peppers, potatoes, corn, wheat, strawberries, citrus fruits, broccoli, soy, melons, and walnuts.

This is just another example of the United States government taking an "innocent until proven guilty" approach to chemicals, allowing most to enter and stay on the market without adequate safety testing. It is only after a problem is found, often after years or even decades of widespread use and accumulation of a vast amount of evidence of harm, that chemicals are banned. In fact, the EPA has only banned nine chemicals in its twenty-seven-year existence. Other countries employ a precautionary principle, which states that if an action has a suspected risk of causing harm to the public or to the environment, in the absence of scientific consensus that it is not harmful, the burden of proof that it is not harmful should fall on those taking action. In other words, the manufacturers of the chemical should prove that it is safe, instead of waiting for an overwhelming amount of evidence that it causes harm while allowing long-term potential toxic exposures to occur. In the name of progress, the US tends to shoot first and ask questions later, protecting the interests of corporations over the health of its citizens.

To avoid the most highly pesticide contaminated fruits and vegetables, consult the Environmental Working Group's (EWG) "Dirty Dozen" list,[2] which is updated yearly, and choose organic for these foods. For instance, strawberries topped the list again this past year with twenty pesticides found in a single sample! If cost is an issue, the EWG also puts out a "Clean 15" list, which identifies produce with lower pesticide residue, and you can focus your organic efforts on the Dirty Dozen while being more relaxed about the Clean 15. Other economical ways to get fresh organic produce are to visit your local farmer's market, join a Community Supported Agriculture (CSA) group, or grow your own. Groups such as ripenearme.com also facilitate sharing of home grown foods. As an added benefit, if you choose locally-grown foods, you will also reduce the carbon footprint of transporting foods sometimes thousands of miles. See the resources section for details on finding organic produce.

Aside from avoiding pesticides, choosing certified organic produce also indicates that it has not been grown with synthetic fertilizers, sewage sludge (which can contain heavy metals and other contaminants), genetically modified organisms (GMOs), or ionizing radiation. Organic dairy, meat, and eggs are raised without use of hormones, antibiotics, or

---

[2] See www.ewg.org/foodnews to download the app or print out a wallet-guide.

GMO-feed and must have access to the outdoors. Look for the USDA Organic label.

Regardless of whether or not produce is organic, wash it before eating. If you can't get organic produce, the benefits of eating fruits and vegetables outweigh the risks of pesticide exposure, so you should still eat plenty of them. Here are some tips that can help to reduce the exposure to pesticides in nonorganic produce:

- **Soak bell peppers, apples, and celery in a solution of 10 percent white vinegar and 90 percent water for ten to twenty-five minutes and then scrub with a vegetable brush for about sixty seconds. Drain and rinse.**
- **After washing, remove the skin from apples, pears, nectarines, peaches, and potatoes.**
- **Soak grapes and cherries in 10 percent white vinegar and 90 percent water solution for sixty minutes. Drain and rinse well.**

3. Eat Real Foods, Not Frankenfoods

Even as a medical student back in the 1990s, I was often asked what diet a person should follow. My simple answer was what I called "The Perimeter Diet"—shop mostly at the perimeter of the store and avoid going down the aisles. The outside lanes of the grocery store are where you will find real, whole foods: fresh vegetables and fruits; nuts, seeds, and unprocessed whole grains; and fresh meat, dairy, poultry, and eggs. These foods come as nature has packaged them, so you don't need a label to identify what's in it. The center aisles of most grocery stores are where you find "Frankenfoods"—food-like substances that normally would not occur in nature. These are highly processed packaged foods that may contain additives, preservatives, artificial colors, artificial sweeteners, chemicals, and fortified nutrients (because processing strips the nutrients from the foods they cleverly add them back in to make the food appear nutritious). Many people have reactions to these substances and the body may recognize these molecules as something other than food. The Frankenfood group also includes GMOs.

Currently, nine foods are from high-GMO crops: soy, corn, cotton (used for cottonseed oil), canola, sugar from sugar beets, zucchini, yellow squash, and papaya grown in Hawaii or China. Alfalfa, which is used for hay for animal feed, is also high-GMO. This technology was developed to create plants that are more resistant to weeds, pests, and other diseases, improve crop yield, and make produce more shelf stable. Unfortunately, many of these promises have not borne out: the weeds and pests become resistant to herbicides and pesticides and crop yields have not really improved. Meanwhile, many scientists and consumers have developed concern about the use of GMO foods. Why? One reason is that when these foods are genetically modified, they are designed with a new gene inserted into them that was never part of the natural makeup. The inserted gene may be from a virus, bacteria, plant, or animal. When the gene is inserted, mutations can develop in the DNA of the recipient plant (or animal) that can alter its health properties. In addition, many of these crops have been engineered to be resistant to herbicides sprayed during the growing phase, allowing more chemicals like glyphosate to be sprayed without damaging the crop.

How do GMOs Relate to Glyphosate?

Glyphosate is a broad-spectrum organophosphate systemic herbicide used to kill weeds that compete with crops and as a ripening agent to assist with harvesting. Since the 1990s, the amount of glyphosate being used in the United States and worldwide has skyrocketed as has the frequency of application. It gets absorbed into the plants that we eat and has been found to disrupt the cytochrome P450 enzyme system, which is a major part of our detoxification process. Research also suggests that glyphosate may have other adverse health effects due to its actions as a mineral chelator (binding key minerals that are essential to health), endocrine disrupter (mimicking hormones), mitochondrial poison (depleting energy), and allergen. Even at very low doses, it may cause health effects such as contributing to fatty liver disease. In 2015, the World Health Organization's International Agency for Research on Cancer (IARC) declared glyphosate a "probable human carcinogen" and many countries have banned or are considering banning its use. Among the other controversies around GMO crops and the heavy use of glyphosate are the depletion of soil nutrients by this widespread farming practice, a lack of increase in crop yield, and an increase in resistant "superweeds." In addition, glyphosate contributes to the destruction of beneficial microbes in the soil and the gut.

Glyphosate is sprayed on a range of fruits, nuts, and vegetables (at least seventy food crops) for weed management and is also used as a ripening agent for wheat, rye, rice, barley, and oats. This may be part of the reason why we've seen exponential increases in people with wheat and gluten sensitivities and allergies in recent years. Glyphosate accumulates in leaves, grains, and fruit and cannot be removed by washing or cooking. Residues have been found in foods commonly consumed such as cookies, crackers, boxed cereals, and chips. A 2014 study in the *Journal of Environmental and Analytical Toxicology* found that glyphosate was significantly higher in the urine of people consuming conventionally grown versus organic food. In that same study, those with chronic illnesses had significantly higher glyphosate residues in their urine than the healthy population. And it's not just in our food: because of its widespread and increased use, glyphosate is now contaminating our groundwater and air.

Use of this chemical has increased approximately fifteen-fold since 1994, when genetically modified "Roundup Ready" glyphosate-tolerant crops were introduced, and a longitudinal study published in the *Journal of the American Medical Association* in 2017 showed dramatically increased levels over the last two decades of glyphosate and its metabolite in human samples.

Glyphosate formulations have never been tested for long-term safety, and industry tests have been on glyphosate alone, the presumed "active ingredient". However, formulations sold and used contain many other ingredients known as adjuvants, which are toxic in and of themselves and increase the toxicity of glyphosate. Only the presumed active ingredients are tested and assessed for safety before being released onto the market. Unfortunately, this fundamental flaw in regulatory testing applies to all pesticides worldwide. A 2014 study testing major pesticides in their complete formulations (including Roundup) found that they were up to 1,000 times more toxic to human cells than their isolated active ingredients.

Another way crops such as corn, potato, and cotton (cottonseed oil) have been genetically modified is by adding a gene that produces Bt toxin. Bt toxin kills certain insects by poking holes in the walls of their stomach and intestines. When Bt toxin is sprayed on the plant, it does its job warding off insect damage to crops, and then washes off and is biodegradable. However, when it's genetically inserted into the plant, it can't be washed off and it doesn't biodegrade. We end up, therefore, consuming Bt toxin within the food, and this can have negative human health effects. A 2012 study in the *Journal of Applied Toxicology* showed that Bt toxin can poke holes in human cells in the same way that it kills insects, potentially causing leaky gut and other problems. When a person has leaky gut, the lining of the small intestine does not work properly and substances pass into the bloodstream that normally are kept out. This may result in immune reactions and inflammation that can affect various parts of the body.

Scientists at the Food and Drug Administration (FDA) have suggested that GMO foods could create adverse health effects and requested in-depth, long-term studies; however, none have been conducted to date. Sixty-four countries including Russia, China, and the European Union currently require labeling of GMO foods. But despite more than 90 percent of polled Americans favoring the labeling of GMO foods, Vermont is the only state that currently requires it. Luckily, in 2016 a federal bill nicknamed the Denying Americans the Right to Know (or DARK, as in "keeping us in the dark") Act was stopped in the US Senate after passing in the House of Representatives. It would have eliminated the ability of states to require GMO labeling, prevented the FDA from eventually requiring mandatory labeling, and allowed so-called "natural" foods to contain GMO ingredients without labeling. A mandatory national disclosure standard for GMO foods was signed into law in 2016, however specific details have not yet been determined including what may be excluded from labeling and exactly what information will be disclosed.

Whether or not we choose to eat GMO foods, we deserve the right to know which foods are or aren't GMO. In the last year, genetically-modified apples, potatoes, and salmon have also been approved by the FDA; however, at the time of this writing, they have not yet come on the market. One other thing: GMO crops (corn, soy, and alfalfa) are given to animals as feed, so it's best to look for organic when consuming animal products as well. To reduce or eliminate GMOs from your diet, select foods with the certified non-GMO or USDA certified organic label.

Choose Non-GMO for These Foods

High GMO Crops	Animal Products exposed to GMO-Feed	Processed from GMO Crops
Soy	Eggs	Corn syrup
Corn	Milk	Hydrolyzed vegetable protein
Cotton (Cottonseed Oil)	Meat	Molasses (from sugar beets)
Canola	Honey	Sucrose (from sugar beets)
Sugar (from Sugar Beets)	Seafood	Textured vegetable protein
Zucchini	Gelatin	Flavorings
Yellow Squash		Vitamins
Papaya (from Hawaii		Yeast products
or China)		Microbes
		Enzymes

The Non-GMO Project monitors the development of new genetically engineered products, and they are currently monitoring the following foods because they will likely soon be widely GMO or because of known instances of contamination from GMOs: flax, mustard, rice, wheat, apple, mushroom, pineapple, potato, camelina (false flax), salmon, sugarcane, and tomato. In addition, some crops have a cross-pollination risk with GMO crops including: chard, table beets, rutabaga, Siberian kale, bok choy, mizuna, Chinese cabbage, turnip, rapini, tatsoi, acorn squash, delicata squash, pattypan squash, and pumpkin.

In general, choose foods that are in their natural state and avoid foods that contain chemicals or things that you can't pronounce. If it didn't exist 100 years ago and your great-grandmother wouldn't know what it is, it's probably not good for you. As Michael Pollan, author of *Food Rules* and *The Omnivore's Dilemma*, has said, "If it came from a plant, eat it; if it was made in a plant, don't."

Eat Real Foods, Not Frankenfoods:

- **Eat foods that your great-grandmother would recognize.**
- **Avoid Genetically Modified (GMO) crops by choosing USDA Certified Organic or non-GMO verified foods.**
- **Avoid additives, preservatives, and anything artificial.**
- **Reduce processed and packaged foods.**
- **If you eat packaged foods, read the label and understand what exactly it is you are eating. Usually, the simpler the ingredients, the better.**

4. Plant Versus Animal Protein

It is extremely important to consume a quality source of protein, as the amino acids from proteins are essential for many functions of the body, including detoxification. But what kind of protein should we consume? A large body of evidence points to advantages of a mostly plant-based diet, and it is possible to obtain adequate protein from a variety of non-animal sources. Quinoa, amaranth, buckwheat, millet, beans, legumes, nuts, seeds, mushrooms, and even dark leafy greens (e.g., chard, spinach, watercress, or seaweed) can provide essential amino acids when consumed in a varied diet. Aside from potential health benefits of a plant-based diet, eating lower down on the food chain is also good for the global environment because it reduces agricultural chemicals, antibiotic usage, water requirements, and production of greenhouse gases such as methane.

Eating Animals: What to Look For and What to Avoid

If you choose to consume animal products, avoid processed meat, which the IARC labeled as carcinogenic in 2015.

Processed meat is defined as meat transformed through salting, curing, fermentation, smoking, or other processes to enhance flavor or improve preservation. Examples of processed meat include hot dogs (frankfurters), ham, sausages, corned beef, and beef jerky, as well as canned meat and meat-based preparations and sauces. In the same report, the IARC also labeled red meat as a probable carcinogen with strong evidence for a link to colorectal cancer as well as pancreatic and prostate cancer, so it's wise to at least moderate your intake.

By choosing organic sources of meat, poultry, eggs, and dairy products, you will reduce your exposure to chlorinated pesticides and other toxins such as DDT and PCBs, antibiotics, growth hormones, and high-GMO ingredients. The leading sources of chlorinated pesticides in our diet are from nonorganic beef, nonorganic dairy products, nonorganic butter, farm-raised fish (especially salmon and catfish), and sport fish from contaminated areas. (More on fish in the next section.) Some vegetables may also be contaminated with chlorinated pesticides from the soil, like leafy vegetables, squash, cucumber, and zucchini. Although chlorinated pesticides like DDT have been mostly banned from use in the United States, their persistent presence in the environment poses an ongoing threat to health. These substances can cause mitochondrial toxicity and affect neurological, immunological, and endocrinological systems, although they can also affect the cardiovascular, respiratory, gastrointestinal, and other bodily systems.

It's also important to consider what type of feed was given to the animal. Is the beef or dairy from grass-fed and grass-finished cows? It should be, since they are meant to graze and ruminate rather than eat grain feed made from corn and soy. Evidence has shown that the feed of the animal affects the balance of fatty acids (omega-3 and omega-6) that are in the animal that is then consumed by people. Furthermore, we should consider how this animal was raised and then milked or slaughtered. We know that human physiology is affected by our psychoemotional environment. Crowded, restrictive factory farming practices, such as penning, de-beaking, etc., also affect the animals' stress response and, in turn, their physiology—the molecules of emotion which we then consume. In these confined animal feeding operations, hormones and antibiotics are used generously to increase growth and combat unsanitary conditions. Most factory farm animals live so close to each other that they don't have enough room to turn around. These types of practices also add to environmental stress, with large demands for cropland (half of the world's grain crops are fed to farm animals) and water and the creation of land and water pollutants and greenhouse gases.

We should find out the source of all of our foods and move towards humane animal care and truly sustainable agricultural practices. It's time to stop our disconnection between the food on our plate and our knowledge of its origins. We can protect the planet, farm animals, and people by: reducing the consumption of meat and other animal-based foods; avoiding products from the worst production systems (e.g., switching from conventional to pasture - raised animal products); and replacing meat and other animal-based foods in the diet with plant-based foods.

Ayurvedic Tips for Consuming Dairy

Dairy is one of the most reactive foods, and many people find they cannot tolerate it. If you have allergies, excessive mucous, or autoimmune conditions, I would recommend avoiding dairy at least for one month, if not giving it up completely. (See Action Step 12 for help in figuring out your food sensitivities.) I do not recommend consuming a lot of dairy, but if you do consume dairy, follow these Ayurvedic tips to optimize your digestion of it:

- Drink it warmed, rather than cold.
- Add turmeric, black pepper, cinnamon, or ginger to reduce mucous formation.
- Choose organic, whole, pasture-raised, and non-homogenized milk.
- Consume dairy products alone or with food with a sweet taste to avoid improper food combinations.

What About Meat and Dairy Substitutes?

For those who want to avoid meat, keep meat-substitute products to a minimum because they are highly processed and usually derived from soy, another food to which many people have become reactive. Instead, explore other savory tastes such as mushrooms, sea vegetables, and fermented foods, all of which have beneficial health properties.

There are a range of plant-based "milks" readily available as dairy substitutes. Starbucks even has soy, almond, and coconut milk as options now. Soy milk (if you're not reactive to it) has the best protein profile, containing all of the essential amino acids necessary. If choosing soy, opt for organic or non-GMO and read the label to avoid carrageenan, an additive that may be pro-inflammatory. Hemp milk has great omega-3 fatty acids, is a good source of protein, and may be more digestible and have more nutrient availability than soy milk. Almond milk has some good nutrients like magnesium but does not have as much protein. It's low in calories and contains some heart-healthy fat. Cashew milk is similar in nutritional profile to almond milk. Coconut milk contains beneficial saturated fatty acids and medium-chain triglycerides (MCT), but negligible protein content. Rice milk is very well tolerated but high in natural sugars and low in protein. Many of these dairy substitutes can be made at home with a blender, but store-bought milk substitutes may be fortified with calcium, vitamin D, and other nutrients. If purchasing packaged milk substitutes, avoid canned coconut milk (which may be lined with Bisphenol A [BPA]) as well as products with thickeners, emulsifiers, other additives, and sweeteners.

Now as for cheese, I love it. I love it so much that when I stopped eating cheese for one month (and that was the only change that I made), I lost ten pounds. That's a lot of cheese! So I would love to tell you that there is some awesome cheese substitute out there, but unfortunately I have not found it yet. The one I like currently is an almond-based cheddar cheese—it has decent flavor and melts well. Other nut-based cheeses are also available. (If you know of an awesome non-dairy cheese, let me know please!)

There are non-dairy options for yogurts made from soy, coconut, almond and rice milks. The nutrient values differ; so, again pay attention to the label and know what you are getting in terms of protein and sugar content. Most store-bought yogurts are so full of sugar you might as well eat a candy bar, or they contain artificial sweeteners which are best avoided. You may consider making your own home-made yogurt.

"There is no question that largely vegetarian diets are as healthy as you can get. The evidence is so strong and overwhelming and produced over such a long period of time that it's no longer debatable."
– Marion Nestle, Ph.D., M.P.H., Paulette Goddard Professor, Department of Nutrition, Food Studies, and Public Health, New York University

To Optimize Your Diet (Including Protein):

- **Make the majority of your diet plant-based.**
- **Choose USDA Certified Organic if eating animal products. Avoid direct exposure of meat to an open flame or a hot metal surface and avoid prolonged cooking times (especially at high temperatures) to reduce formation of heterocyclic amines (HCAs) and polycyclic aromatic hydrocarbons (PAHs) which can increase risk of cancer. PAHs can also be formed on other charred foods, including vegetables.**
- **Investigate the source of your animal products, and avoid those from factory farms.**

5. Something Fishy

What happens when we eat big fish like tuna and swordfish? As with any time that we consume higher up the food chain, we eat everything that has accumulated throughout the food chain, including the heavy metal mercury and other pollutants such as polychlorinated biphenyls (PCBs). Here's how it works in the case of mercury: Power plants that burn coal release pollutants including mercury into the air, which settles in the water. Water can also become contaminated with mercury through disposal of auto parts, fluorescent lightbulbs, and medical products. Small plankton and fish in these waters absorb the mercury and cannot clear it from their bodies. Bigger fish absorb and accumulate mercury from the water in addition to the entire mercury load of the smaller fish that they eat, so the highest levels of mercury tend to be in the larger fish. Mercury is known to have harmful effects on the nervous, immune, and digestive systems and can even cause death if exposed to large amounts. Avoid eating fish that have high levels of mercury, such as tuna (particularly albacore, ahi, and bigeye), orange roughy, swordfish, shark, and king mackerel. Mercury leaves the body very slowly (the amount of time it takes for levels to be reduced by half in the brain is twenty years!), and some people have more difficulty processing it out of their bodies than others. In addition to food, the most common source of mercury exposure is from dental filings.

If eating fish, choose smaller fish such as black cod (sable), sardines, and anchovies, which have the least amount of mercury while providing beneficial omega-3 fatty acids. Salmon is touted as the healthiest fish to eat, but be aware of the type of salmon you are getting. Wild Alaskan salmon (coho (silver), Chinook (king), pink (humpback), or red (sockeye)) may be available fresh from June through September and can be purchased frozen or canned throughout the year. Vital Choice is a company that offers canned Alaskan salmon that does not have BPA in the can lining. Steer clear of farmed or Atlantic salmon that is highly contaminated with PCBs, dioxin, other persistent chlorinated contaminants, and artificial dyes. In addition, farmed salmon are fed fishmeal (smaller fish which have also been contaminated with PCBs), fish oils, and GMO soy and corn. Aside from producing poor quality polluted fish, the use of pesticides, antibiotics, and other chemicals in fish farming also pollutes the environment and damages local ecosystems. If you do choose farmed fish, make sure that the fish were:

- **raised without antibiotics or hormones.**
- **farmed in low-density (meaning not cramped) pens or tanks.**
- **not in tanks or pens treated with synthetic herbicides.**
- **fed a more natural diet that does not include genetically-modified plants or land-based foods.**

What are PCBs and PFCs?
PCBs, or polychlorinated biphenyls, were originally manufactured for use as coolants in electrical transformers, but also have served many other industrial uses. Unfortunately,

they are persistent chemicals that bioaccumulate, meaning the amounts build up and accumulate in living things. PCBs have been found in all adults and newborns tested for the substance in the United States and appear in fat samples of people tested all over the world. PCBs cause mitochondrial dysfunction (damage at the cellular level), which affects the immune system, leads to weight gain, and can act as a carcinogen. Children exposed to higher levels of PCBs in utero have more cognitive defects, poorer gross motor function, and less visual memory than those who were less exposed. Adults who ate Great Lakes fish with high PCB levels had neurotoxic effects. Due to these negative health effects, a worldwide ban on PCB production has been in effect since the 1970s. But since they persist in the environment—never going away—they are still in people, animals, fish, and soil all over the world. They are found in high amounts in non-organic butter and farmed salmon and catfish.

PFCs are a family of perfluorinated chemicals that includes perfluorooctanoic acid (PFOA) also known as C8, perfluorooctanesulfonic acid (PFOS), and other per- and polyfluoroalkyl substances (PFASs). These have been used to make products stain-resistant, waterproof, or nonstick (such as Teflon and Scotchguard). They are also used in industries such as aerospace, automotive, construction, and electronics. Both PFOA and PFOS are very persistent in the environment and in the human body, with 98 percent of thousands of human blood samples found to have PFCs in the Center for Disease Control (CDC) 2003–2004 National Health and Nutrition Examination Survey (NHANES). Exposure to PFCs has been linked to obesity, high cholesterol, cancer and tumor growth, and reproductive, developmental, liver, kidney, and immunological effects. Although PFOA and PFOS are no longer manufactured in the United States, they are still produced in other countries and continue to be imported into the US in consumer goods such as carpets, leather and apparel, textiles, paper and packaging, coatings, and rubber and plastics. Other types of PFCs are often found in takeout food containers, pizza boxes, nonstick cookware, popcorn bags, cosmetics, and outdoor and stain-resistant clothing. Because they are so persistent in the environment, people are exposed through air, household dust, soil, water, and contaminated food, including fish. A 2008 FDA study found that PFCs migrate to food during use and that oil and grease significantly increase that effect. The FDA has approved twenty next-generation PFCs for coating paper and paperboard used to serve food. The problem with these new chemicals is that they have not been adequately tested for safety, and scientists are concerned that they have the same effects and persistence as the old compounds. Grease-resistant food contact paper and paperboard free of PFCs have been available for at least ten years and can be used as alternatives.

In May 2016, more than 200 scientists from 40 countries signed the Madrid Statement, warning about the harms of fluorochemicals and calling for action to eliminate their use. The EPA strengthened its advisory for PFOAs and PFOSs in drinking water at that time, and since then, a number of states have taken steps to develop drinking water guidelines, but these substances are still present in many everyday products.

Choosing Safer Fish:
- **Avoid eating fish which have high levels of mercury, including swordfish, shark, orange roughy, king mackerel, and tuna.**
- **Tuna is the most common source of mercury exposure in the United States. Limit consumption of tuna to less than two servings per week and stick to light or skipjack tuna, which have less mercury. Children should avoid albacore tuna, which has more mercury,**

and women of childbearing age should eat no more than four ounces per week.

- **Choose smaller fish such as black cod (sable), sardines, and anchovies, which have the least amount of mercury while providing beneficial omega-3 fatty acids. Crab, scallops, and shrimp are also low mercury.**
- **Use the NRDC** "Mercury in Fish" **or EWG's** "Consumers Guide to Seafood" **to help choose lower mercury fish and avoid high mercury fish.**
- **Sushi lovers can reduce mercury exposure by choosing eel, salmon, crab, and clam which are lower in mercury.**
- **Use** Monterey Bay Aquarium's Seafood Watch **app for sustainable seafood recommendations (this does not comment on mercury).**

6. Drink Good Clean Water

Water makes up about 60 to 80 percent of the human body. It is essential to life, and we need to take in enough daily from water, other liquids, and food to replace the amount that is lost in urine, stool, breathing, and evaporation from our skin. Our body needs water for digestion, absorption, circulation, transportation of nutrients, excretion of waste products, lubrication and protection of joints and our nervous system, and maintenance of body temperature. Studies show that even mild dehydration can impair many aspects of brain function.

You can tell when you're getting enough fluids by looking at your urine. When you're well hydrated, urine flows freely and is light in color and virtually free of odor. When you're not getting enough fluids, the kidneys will hold onto more and concentrate the urine, which increases color and odor. In addition, fluids are reabsorbed in the colon, and if we are dehydrated, it may contribute to constipation. Water losses increase in warmer climates, at higher altitudes, and with intense physical activity, as well as with illnesses resulting in fever, diarrhea, or vomiting.

Drinking fresh, pure water is best, but other fluids (other than alcohol and caffeinated beverages) also help replenish our internal fluid balance. Choosing water instead of sugar-sweetened beverages saves money, reduces the risk for dental cavities, helps with weight management, and reduces sugar swings. About 20 percent of our fluid intake comes from foods, particularly from fruits and vegetables that have a high water content such as celery, tomatoes, and melons.

How to Get Clean Water

The best way to get pure, clean water is to avoid drinking out of plastic and make sure your water is filtered to remove contaminants. Although plastic water bottles can make drinking water more convenient, studies have shown that the plastic can also leach into the drinking water. (See Action Step 14 for more information about plastics.) Many bottled waters have been found to contain other contaminants, and about 40 percent of bottled waters are nothing more than packaged tap water. Despite marketing hype, bottled water is not necessarily any safer or better than tap water, and it can cost up to 1,900 times more! Bottled water may also be contaminated with plastic that leaches from the bottles, especially when heated. Plastic water bottles are also bad for our environment, with Americans throwing away about fifty million bottles every day. Instead, fill reusable glass bottles or stainless steel containers with your favorite water. Bottled water may be the best option in some situations, however, such as when tap water is unsafe for consumption or when water is needed to make infant formula and available tap water contains fluoride. If using bottled water to make infant formula, use water that's fluoride-free to reduce the risk of fluorosis (see Action Step 36 for more on fluoride).

If you receive municipal water, you can check tap water quality by viewing your local water company's annual report and by checking EWG's Tap Water Database. Those who use well water or who want additional water testing can request testing through a private lab. To find a lab, call the EPA Safe Drinking Water Hotline or find state certified programs and laboratories on the EPA website.

Many of the 250-plus contaminants detected in tap water are at levels that are legal under the Safe Drinking Water Act or state regulations, but well above levels found to pose health risks including cancer, neurologic damage, fertility problems, developmental harm to children or fetuses, and hormonal disruption. Some of the contaminants of concern include chromium-6 or hexavalent chromium (the industrial chemical that Erin Brockovich found was making people sick in Hinkley, California), lead, PFCs, microplastics, nitrates, industrial solvents, and pharmaceuticals.

To improve your water quality, use a filtration and purification system. Depending on your needs, you can choose from various filter types: pitcher/large-dispenser, faucet-mounted, faucet-integrated, on-counter, under-sink, refrigerator, and whole-house filters. Activated carbon filters are economical and are available as pitcher, tap-mounted, and large-dispenser types. But effectiveness varies widely. Some remove only chlorine, while others remove contaminants such as lead, mercury, and volatile organic compounds (VOCs). Activated carbon does not remove arsenic, fluoride, hexavalent chromium, nitrate, or perchlorate. When looking at activated charcoal filters, look for coconut shell carbon, which is better than standard carbon "charcoal" filtering media for removing chlorine and VOCs. Carbon block filters may be more effective than granular, due to increased surface area. A more expensive reverse osmosis (RO) filter is required to remove smaller toxins, such as arsenic, nitrates, hexavalent chromium, fluoride, trichloroethylene, and perchlorate. RO will also remove viral particles and radiation. RO does not remove chlorine, trihalomethanes, or VOCs, therefore many RO systems include an activated carbon component to remove additional contaminants from your water. If choosing a RO filter, get the highest rejection rate that you can afford to maximize the percentage of total dissolved solids (TDS) removed. The most expensive option is a whole-house filter, which will also remove contaminants such as chlorinated compounds from your shower. Shower-head filters are an economical option but fail to remove chloramines. (See Action Step 36 for information on shower-head and whole-house filters and a discussion on chlorination and fluoridation of water.) Make sure to maintain your filter and purifier regularly to keep the level of effectiveness consistently high.

Tips to Stay Hydrated with Clean Water:
- **Keep a bottle of water with you in your car, at your desk, or in your bag, preferably a reusable glass or stainless container rather than a plastic bottle. Skip aluminum, which can contain a lining with BPA.**
- **If you like flavor, add slices of lemon, lime, oranges, cucumber, fresh mint, or a few fresh berries to your water.**
- **Gotta have some fizz? Mix sparkling water (which can also help alkalinize your urine) with a small amount of berry juice.**
- **Don't reuse single-use bottled water bottles. The plastic can harbor bacteria and break down to release plastic chemicals, especially if heated.**
- **Determine what contaminants are in your water supply and then get a water purifier to handle the contaminants. Change filters as recommended.**

What the Frack?

With less than 1 percent of freshwater accessible for drinking on our planet, water is one of our most valuable resources, and yet we don't necessarily treat it as such. We run our sinks and showers too long, we hose things down, we wash our cars, we keep beautiful green lawns, we support water-wasting agricultural and industrial practices. While traveling in India, one person said to me, "You Americans have so much clean water, you pee and poop in it." Here is yet another area where Americans tend to be overconsumers. These practices are wasteful, of course, but what's even more upsetting is that we allow our valuable clean groundwater supplies to be wasted and poisoned by fracking.

Fracking, or hydraulic fracturing, is a technique to recover difficult-to-reach gas and oil from shale rock. Fracking involves drilling down into the earth and directing a high-pressure mixture of water, sand, and chemicals at the rock to release the gas inside. While fracking in the United States has significantly boosted domestic oil production, it has also created a glut since 2014. Although this resulted in cheaper gas prices, a significant environmental cost comes along with this practice. Fracking uses huge amounts of water to liberate the gas and contaminates groundwater with potentially carcinogenic chemicals and methane, which is highly flammable. In addition, propane, methane, and ethane in the air near the wells can lead to respiratory problems as well as contribute to climate change. There are also concerns that the fracking process can cause small earth tremors and that surface spills may contaminate the surrounding soil. A newly released study found 6,648 spills in just four states over the past ten years. A variety of other health problems may also be associated with fracking including asthma, migraines, fatigue, sinusitis, problems in pregnancy, contamination of drinking wells and air with carcinogens, and other concerns.

Although companies could be fined if they are found to be polluting drinking water under the Clean Water Act, the

Energy Policy Act of 2005 exempted runoff from gas and oil activities. In addition, the Energy Policy Act included a loophole exempting fracking fluids (other than diesel fuels) from the Safe Drinking Water Act, which otherwise would regulate how contaminants are injected underground. These federal exemptions leave our water supplies unprotected from fracking, leading individual municipalities to ban fracking one-by-one on their own. However, at the time of this writing, the state of Florida has been moving forward with a bill that would take away even the ability of local municipalities to ban fracking. This is another example of our dependence on fossil fuels causing damage to our health and our environment.

7. The Truth About Sugar, Sweeteners, and Diet Drinks

Sugary drinks like soda, fruit punch, lemonade, sports and energy drinks, and other sugar-sweetened beverages can contribute to obesity, diabetes, and fatty liver disease. Although it may have more nutrients, even fruit juice is on the sugary-drink list, containing as much sugar (albeit as naturally occurring fruit sugar or fructose) and calories as soft drinks and lacking beneficial fiber that you get from eating whole fruit. The average can of sugar-sweetened soda or fruit punch provides about 150 calories, almost all of them from sugar and usually in the form of high-fructose corn syrup. That's the equivalent of ten teaspoons of table sugar! In terms of detoxification, excessive sugar impairs the Phase I detoxification pathway in the liver, reducing the ability to clear toxic compounds from the bloodstream.

But the surprising news for many is that substituting sugary drinks with diet drinks is not necessarily the solution. Recent studies have shown that people who drink diet soda gained weight and gained more abdominal fat that those who didn't drink diet soda. There are a few hypotheses of how this may happen. A recent study in mice showed that artificial sweeteners actually changed the gut bacteria of mice in ways that made them vulnerable to insulin resistance and glucose intolerance, both of which can lead to weight gain. Other research suggests that artificial sweeteners are associated with a drop in the hormone leptin, which inhibits hunger. And because artificial sweeteners are thousands of times sweeter than regular sugar, our taste buds become more accustomed to a sweet taste without the feedback of calories or satiation, potentially causing increased food consumption. The point is that drinking sweetened beverages, no matter how they are sweetened—sugar, fruit juice, high-fructose corn syrup, or artificial sweeteners—is just not good for you.

Rethink Your Drink:

- **Drink a glass of water first.** We often reach for our favorite beverage or food when we are actually thirsty. See if replenishing your fluids does the trick without adding unnecessary sugar or chemicals.
- **Try other beverages such as plain tea or sparkling water.** Add a slice of lemon, lime, or cucumber, a sprig of mint, or a few berries for flavor if needed. A *small* amount of sugar, honey, or stevia during your transition-from-soda phase is ok. The important thing is that you are aware and in charge of exactly what's going into your drink.
- **Buy caffeine-free.** If you drink a lot of soda and are not quite ready to give it up, switch to a caffeine-free version. When your body gets used to consuming caffeine, you crave more of it, so stop this part of the feedback loop and you might find it easier to quit.
- **Save it for special occasions.** Shifting from doing something every day to only doing it on occasion will drastically reduce its impact.
- **Avoid or preempt triggers.** Do you always get soda with a certain food? Try different foods that you don't normally associate with a sweetened beverage. Or try

an unsweetened beverage such as iced tea or lemon water. Do you refill all day at the office? Bring your own healthy beverage or refillable water bottle.

- **Switch to a brand with fewer artificial ingredients and without high-fructose corn syrup.** These generally contain less sugar than the major brands, and since they cost more, you might be more apt to think of them as a special treat.

So, drinking sweet stuff is not good for you. How about eating it? From an Ayurvedic perspective, the sweet taste is one of the six fundamental tastes and provides nourishment to your body, mind, and spirit (see Action Step 15 for a discussion of all six tastes). We get it in a variety of forms—beyond foods we typically think of as sweets like pastries and ice cream, the sweet taste is found in fruit, starchy vegetables, grains, nuts, seeds, and animal and fish sources. Because these foods are so nourishing, people tend to crave the sweet taste. Food manufacturers know this and produce foods that appeal to our sweet cravings, leading us to consume more added sugar than ever before. Americans consume about twenty teaspoons of added sugar (in the form of various sweeteners) every day, according to a report from the 2005–2010 National Health and Nutrition Examination Survey (NHANES) database. Since it is well known that eating too much sugar can bring you out of balance and lead to major health issues, including diabetes, heart disease, and liver disease, many health-conscious folks wonder which alternative sweetener would be best to satisfy our tastes. To answer this question, you first need to look at how your body metabolizes three major forms of sugar: glucose, fructose, and sucrose.

Glucose (also known as dextrose) is the most basic sugar molecule and is the body's preferred fuel. Most carbohydrates that you eat are broken down into glucose, which your body uses for immediate energy or stores for later use in your muscle or liver. Your body needs blood sugar levels to stay in a certain range, and the hormone insulin helps regulate these levels. When the body has problems managing insulin and can no longer regulate blood sugar levels, diabetes develops.

Fructose is another simple sugar that is naturally found in fruits. It is sweeter than glucose and sucrose and is a marker of the ripeness and nutritional density of fruit. Processed sweeteners such as agave nectar and high-fructose corn syrup contain varying amounts of fructose, but due to the processing, these provide the sweet taste and calories stripped of beneficial nutrients and fiber found in whole fruits. While eating whole fruits can be beneficial, excessive consumption of processed fructose can have some negative effects. Fructose is lipogenic, which means that it is quickly turned into fat. Almost all of the fructose you ingest is metabolized in the liver, and much of it is stored as fat and glycogen. This can contribute to elevated triglycerides (a type of fat in your blood that can raise the risk of heart disease) and nonalcoholic fatty liver disease (an accumulation of fat in the liver that can cause inflammation and scarring). Another drawback to fructose is that, unlike glucose, it doesn't activate the feedback mechanism that curbs your appetite when you eat, potentially leading to overeating. It's best to eat fructose in the form of whole fruits and honey where the wholeness of the food prevents overeating and to avoid consumption of concentrated sweeteners such as agave nectar and high-fructose corn syrup, especially in sweetened beverages.

Sucrose is a combination of glucose and fructose and is commonly found in table sugar made from sugarcane or sugar beets. It's also found in corn and other plants. When you eat sucrose, your body breaks it down into individual molecules of fructose and glucose.

Here's the lowdown on some of the most common types of sweeteners.

These are basically sugar:

- **White Sugar:** This sweet crystalline substance is mainly extracted from sugarcane or sugar beets and gets its sweetness from sucrose, which is broken down by the body into an even ratio of glucose (50 percent) and fructose (50 percent). Note: If the label on a sugar package doesn't say the product comes from sugarcane, then most likely it comes from sugar beets, which are a heavily genetically modified food. I advise everyone to avoid GMO foods, so if buying sugar choose USDA Certified Organic or non-GMO product verified.
- **Evaporated Cane Juice:** Made from fresh sugarcane juice that is evaporated and then crystallized, this has no added benefit over table sugar other than a slight flavor difference and some trace minerals.
- **Molasses:** This thick syrup is the by-product when sugarcane is processed to make refined sugar. Blackstrap molasses has a bittersweet taste and contains minerals and nutrients such as iron, calcium, manganese, copper, and potassium. One tablespoon provides 12.2 grams of sugar (just slightly less than table sugar) and converts to glucose more slowly than table sugar.
- **Coconut Sugar/Coconut Palm Sugar:** Made from the sap of the coconut palm, it has the same calories and carbohydrates as table sugar. It is dark like brown sugar, which is a partially refined sugar that contains some amount of molasses, and has a similar taste. Coconut sugar has been touted in the press recently for containing 70 to 79 percent sucrose, and only 3 to 9 percent fructose and glucose. However, since sucrose breaks down in the body in a 1 to 1 ratio of fructose to glucose, coconut sugar actually contains between 38 percent to 50 percent fructose, and thus may not be much better

than table sugar. Some brands may mix coconut sugar with cane sugar and other ingredients.

- **Palm Sugar/Date Palm Sugar/Palm Sugar:** Made by pulverizing dates into a powder, this is less processed and contains all of the nutrients found in dates, including potassium, magnesium, and calcium. Palm sugar clumps and doesn't melt, so it's not a great substitute for white sugar, but may be a good substitute in some recipes calling for brown sugar. It is often used in Southeast Asian and Indian cooking.

These may have some health benefits but have higher fructose levels:

- **Honey:** Consists of glucose and up to 40 to 50 percent fructose (ranges vary), and it has antioxidants and trace amounts of vitamins and minerals. While raw or unrefined honey has a glycemic index of about 30, processed honey can be much higher, meaning it is converted more rapidly to glucose and can spike blood sugars. Processed honey is also stripped of the nutrients contained in raw or unrefined honey. In Ayurveda, honey is viewed as the best sweetener and is used medicinally as well as in food. According to Ayurveda, honey should never be cooked. Do not give honey to children under one year of age to reduce risk of infant botulism.
- **Maple Syrup:** Extracted from the sap of a maple tree, different grades of maple syrup relate to the darkness of the syrup, and the darker ones have a stronger maple flavor. It contains some minerals, including manganese, zinc, iron, calcium, and potassium, as well as antioxidants (darker syrups have higher antioxidant levels). Maple syrup consists of about 65 percent sucrose and

has less fructose than honey. I enjoy using small amounts of grade-B maple syrup as a sweetener in my cooking. Grade B contains more minerals and has a more robust maple flavor than grade A.

A possible decent alternative if you choose correctly:

- **Stevia:** Extracted from a plant called *Stevia rebaudiana*, this sweetener comes as a less processed green leaf form or a more processed white, powdery substance or liquid. There are differences between these forms with the less processed being about 30 times sweeter and the more processed about 200 times sweeter than table sugar. While stevia has zero calories and doesn't affect glucose or insulin levels, be mindful of the amount that you use. Just one teaspoon of liquid stevia is equivalent in sweetness to a whole cup of sugar. I have not yet come across any brain studies of stevia, but I suspect that the super sweetness without the caloric messaging to your brain to signal fullness might cause you to crave more sweet foods. Stevia can be used in baking. Some of the stevia products found in many grocery stores contain other ingredients such as erythritol and dextrose (which is actually a form of glucose), so read your labels and make sure you're buying the best source if using this sweetener—look for green leaf stevia.

These are worse than sugar or can produce side effects:

- **Agave Nectar and Syrup:** Higher in fructose than high-fructose corn syrup, agave nectar is on my list of health-food imposters. In the agave plant, most of the sweetness comes from a type of fructose called inulin, a fiber that has some health benefits. However, the inulin is processed into a syrup that has a fructose content estimated to be as high as 90 percent without the benefit of the fiber. As a comparison, the much-maligned high-fructose corn syrup has about 55 percent fructose.

- **Brown Rice Syrup:** Processed from brown rice, this syrup is no health food either and may even contain gluten as well as arsenic. It is often added to foods such as cereal, protein bars, and baby formulas.

- **Sugar Alcohols:** These naturally occur in foods and are sometimes used as sugar substitutes in many "sugar-free" products such as candies, gum, and many processed foods. Examples include xylitol, sorbitol, and erythritol. Sugar alcohols contain 1/2 to 1/3 fewer calories than table sugar and are not as sweet as sugar. Some forms may not spike blood sugar and insulin levels because they are not digested easily. However, this also leads to potential side effects such as gas, bloating, and diarrhea.

- **Artificial Sweeteners:** Sucralose, aspartame, and saccharin get their sweetness from chemicals other than the three sugars of glucose, fructose, and sucrose. While they may be low- or no calorie, they have no nutritional benefits and should be avoided.

So, which sweetener is best? In reality, there isn't much difference between white table sugar and other natural sweeteners, including coconut sugar, honey, maple syrup, and molasses. To the body they are all sugar to be converted to glucose for metabolic fuel.

What's the important take-home point? Too much sweet, in any form, brings the body-mind connection out of balance. Eating more food—of any kind—than you need will push your body into storage mode and create a variety of health issues. Therefore, all forms of sweets are best in moderation.

Tips to Help Break a Sweet Habit:

- Beware of added sugars in processed foods, even in so-called healthy foods such as protein bars and yogurt.
- Avoid artificial sweeteners.
- Reduce the amount of sugary-sweet foods you consume. Desserts should be an occasional treat and not a daily event. When you do indulge, choose a treat with high-quality ingredients and savor the experience. As you reduce the amount of added sugars you consume, you will need less to appreciate the sweet taste.
- Eat less packaged and processed foods which often contain added sugar.
- Read labels: If an ingredient ends in –ose, (as in sucrose or dextrose), it is a form of sugar. Other ingredients to be aware of that essentially mean sugar: any type of nectar, sugar, juice, or syrup, agave, barley malt, dextrin, dextran, diatase, diatastic malt, honey, maltodextrin, and turbinado.
- If you have a sugar addiction, you may need to eliminate sugar for a period of time to stop the cycle.

8. The Skinny on Fats

Fats are essential to our health. They are burned as fuel for our body and are an integral part of our cell membranes. Fats are essential for healthy skin, hair, and brain function and play an important role in regulating inflammation, mood, and behavior. Some fats are absolutely necessary for the proper functioning of the body and must be eaten because they're not manufactured by the body. These are called essential fatty acids (EFAs) and include omega-3 alpha-linolenic acid and omega-6 linoleic acid found in vegetable oils, nuts, seeds, leafy greens, fish, and grass-fed animal products.

Omega-3 fatty acids are among the most important essential fatty acids for health and many people have a deficiency.

Oil from cold-water fish (salmon, herring, sardines, mackerel, and krill) is the highest source of the anti-inflammatory omega-3s eicosapentaenoic acid (EPA) and docosahexaenoic acid (DHA). Algae-based supplements can also be a source of EPA and DHA in lesser amounts. While nuts, seeds, and some vegetables (flax, chia, walnuts, Brazil nuts, winter squash, leafy greens, cauliflower, broccoli, Brussels sprouts, and beans, such as split black lentils or urad dahl, French beans, navy beans, and soybeans) can provide omega-3s in the form of alpha-linolenic acid (ALA), the effects are less potent than the other fatty acids. Even though the body can convert some ALA to EPA and DHA, the amounts produced are very limited.

For a long time, saturated fats were thought to contribute to heart disease, but recent studies have found that it is not the consumption of saturated fats in general, but the specific source of these fats that can make a difference. Saturated fats from cheese, butter, and beef fat tend to increase inflammatory compounds and lead to heart disease, while saturated fats from sources such as coconut, chocolate, nuts, and seeds have some health benefits.

Monounsaturated fats are a type of fat that helps reduce "bad" cholesterol levels and also provides nutrients such as vitamin E, which is an important antioxidant. Sources include olive oil, canola oil, avocados, peanut butter and peanut oil, and many nuts and seeds including safflower and sesame oils.

The demonization of fats has perhaps come to an end. In fact, many people are now eating fat to get thin. In Ayurveda, a cleansing process known as Panchakarma employs copious amounts of oil both internally and externally to help flush the system. (Please note that this procedure should be administered by an experienced professional.) Many of our toxins are stored long-term in fat, so the use of copious amounts of uncontaminated oils can help to move those fat-soluble toxins out. A study of Panchakarma procedures conducted in 2002 at Maharishi University showed that nearly all of the toxins measured, including PCBs and pesticides, were reduced by this detoxification method. Use of non-absorbable consumed oils can also lower levels of toxins such as PCBs.

The one type of fat still considered harmful to our health is trans fats. These fats are found in margarine, vegetable shortening, and partially hydrogenated vegetable oils and should be avoided. The structure of these fats is changed through processing to make them solid at room temperature. Our bodies don't know how to use this fat and can't use it as fuel. Trans fats raise your "bad" low density lipoprotein (LDL) cholesterol levels and lower your "good" high density lipoprotein (HDL) cholesterol levels. Eating trans fats increases your risk of developing heart disease, stroke, and type 2 diabetes. In addition to chemically synthesized trans fats, small amounts of trans fats occur naturally in some meat and dairy products, including beef, lamb, and butterfat. There haven't been enough studies to determine if naturally occurring trans fats have the same negative health effects as those that are manufactured.

Which Fats Should I Eat?

It's important to consume healthy fats from a variety of sources such as avocado, olive, and coconut, as well as from other nuts and seeds. Make sure the oils, nuts, and seeds you consume are not rancid, as this can cause oxidative damage to cells, proteins, and DNA. Antioxidants such as vitamin E are added to most oils to prevent rancidity if they don't already contain natural antioxidants. Most olive oils are stored in dark bottles to reduce the amount of light that reaches the oil, which can also cause it to become rancid. Make sure to check expiration dates and purchase the amount that you intend to consume before the product expires. If you're a fish-eater, choose fatty fish such as wild Alaskan salmon, sardines, herring, flounder, or sole. If you eat animals, consume omega-3 rich eggs, small amounts of grass-fed beef, and small amounts of full-fat dairy from grass-fed cows. Since toxins bioaccumulate in the fat of animals as well as humans, pay attention to where your beef, dairy, poultry, and fish come from and choose organic, humane, and sustainable sources. If you're a vegan, consider taking a plant-based EPA and DHA supplement from algae to get the full range of omega-3 fatty acids.

Tips on Getting Healthy Fats:
- **Choose healthy fats from a variety of sources.**
- **Consume essential fatty acids including omega-3 and omega-6 oils found in vegetables, nuts, seeds, fish, and animal products.**
- **If consuming fish or animals, pay attention to sourcing, and choose organic and less polluted sources.**
- **Saturated fats from coconut, chocolate, nuts, and seeds have health benefits and can be consumed in moderation.**
- **Saturated fats from cheese, butter, and beef fat may lead to inflammation and should be reduced.**
- **Include sources of monounsaturated fats such as olive oil and avocados.**
- **Avoid trans fats that are found in margarine, vegetable shortening, and partially hydrogenated vegetable oils. These are also found in a lot of processed foods.**

9. Give us this Day Our Daily Fiber

As mentioned in Chapter 2, elimination through stool (aka poop) is a major way that toxins leave our body. Fiber is an important part of this equation and plays a role in digestive health, heart disease, diabetes, weight management, and cancer. Most people today don't get enough fiber. Our detox process evolved when we were eating 100 to 150 grams of fiber per day as compared with the average now of 15 to 20 grams per day in the typical Western diet. Adding to another reason why a plant-based diet is beneficial, fiber is found only in foods that come from plants. Foods such as meat, fish, and dairy products don't contain any fiber.

There are two different types of fiber, and each helps the body in different ways, so it is important to get both. **Soluble fiber** soaks up water and is turned into a gel during digestion, helping with digestion and elimination. Sources include oats, barley, nuts, seeds, beans, lentils, peas, flaxseeds, rye, and some fruits and vegetables. It is also found in psyllium, which is a common fiber supplement and can help manage cholesterol. **Insoluble fiber** adds bulk to the stool without being broken down, helping bind and remove toxins through the gut. Sources include bran (wheat, brown rice), nuts, seeds, cereals, vegetables, and the seeds and skins of fruit. Rice bran fiber, in particular, has been shown to increase the excretion of toxins including PCBs and dioxin. Whole grain brown rice will naturally have rice bran fiber. While most people get about 15 grams of fiber in their diet per day, it is recommended that men consume 38 grams and women consume 25 grams per day. If you're needing more, increase your fiber consumption gradually over the course of about two weeks. Avoid wheat bran, as many people are reactive or become constipated with it. Drink plenty of water. When increasing your fiber intake, there may be increase in gas, bloating, and more stool. Decrease the dosage if this does not improve after three days. If you have a digestive issue such as Irritable Bowel Syndrome (IBS) or Small Intestinal Bacterial Overgrowth (SIBO), you may need to modify the amount and type of fiber in your diet.

To encourage regular bowel movements, try the following:

- **Consume plenty of fiber**.
- **Drink plenty of fluids**. The main job of the colon is to reabsorb liquids if we are deficient. Inadequate fluid intake often results in constipation as well as recycling of toxins, so make sure to stay hydrated. See Action Step 6 for details on clean water.

- **Move your body.** Physical activity is not only good for your physique, it also helps facilitate digestion. See Action Step 28 for tips on balanced physical activity. Certain yoga postures can help facilitate digestion and elimination.
- **Go first thing in the morning.** To facilitate a morning bowel movement, drink a cup of warm water with a squeeze of lemon juice upon rising.
- **Allow yourself time**. If we are constantly on the go, then we might not have the time to "go." Relax and try to have the intention of things moving down and out.
- **Position yourself well.** It's only in fairly recent times that we have had a "throne" to sit on while doing our business. For millennia, the routine was to squat, and it still is in many cultures. With this in mind, some clever person designed the Squatty Potty, an add-on little stool to help you to be in more of a squatting position while still using a modern toilet. Alternatively, you can position a small step stool in front of the commode to facilitate this positioning.
- **Consider taking probiotics**. I have seen many patients whose digestive troubles normalized after taking supplemental probiotics. Probiotics that contain beneficial *Bifidobacterium* and *Lactobacillus* species seem to be the most effective. Look for a product with multiple strains and take at least ten billion colony-forming units per day. For further details about probiotics, see Action Step 18.
- **Consider taking Triphala**. Literally meaning three fruits, Triphala is an Ayurvedic formulation of Amalaki (*Emblica offinicalis*), Harataki (*Terminalia chebula*), and Bibhitaki (*Terminalia belerica*) that is used as a bowel tonic and can help greatly with digestion and elimination. Doses range from 500 mg to several grams taken once or twice daily.

- **Use laxatives infrequently.** Stimulant laxatives can lead to dependency if used chronically. These include senna, cascara, bisacodyl, aloe vera gel, and castor oil, which may be found in over-the-counter formulas and in some digestive teas. When used occasionally (less than once per month) they shouldn't cause harm, but if you have a persistent issue, seek care from a qualified healthcare practitioner who can literally get you moving in the right direction.
- **Colonic irrigations.** At times, further cleansing of the colon may be needed. In Ayurveda, we use herbalized oil- or water-based enemas to facilitate detoxification as well as administer herbal treatments. Colon hydrotherapy or colonics may also be helpful. A number of my patients experienced drastic improvements in their health after receiving a series of individually prescribed colonics to remove accumulated toxins. To find a qualified colon hydrotherapist, please see the Resources section.

10. Love Your Liver

As described in Chapter 4, the liver is the main organ for handling toxins, so optimizing your liver function is key. The liver's work of detoxifying uses up and depletes nutrients, and if you don't have enough nutrients to support the process, you can become more vulnerable to the effects of toxins. You can be sure to get all of your nutrients by eating a rainbow of whole foods, clean protein, and savory herbs and spices.

Support liver function by making sure you have these key nutrients:

- **Protein:** A complete mix of essential amino acids from protein sources is needed for proper liver functioning, particularly for phase I detoxification. See Action Step 4 for a discussion on plant and animal protein.
- **Vitamin A (carotenoids):** Choose orange and yellow vegetables like carrots and winter squash, spinach and

other leafy greens, and tomatoes. Vitamin A is a fat-soluble vitamin and is best absorbed when consumed with healthy fat in a meal.

- **Vitamin B6**: Good sources include wild salmon, potato, sweet potato, turkey, avocado, chicken, beef, sunflower seeds, spinach, banana, cabbage, pinto beans, and lentils.

- **Vitamin B9 (folate):** Green leafy vegetables are rich sources of folate and provide the basis for its name (think foliage). Asparagus, broccoli, beets, lentils, legumes, papaya, and avocado are also excellent sources.

- **Vitamin B12:** Sources for this essential nutrient are animal products, such as meat, poultry, fish (including shellfish), and to a lesser extent dairy products and eggs. Although cremini mushrooms are a source of B12, one cup provides you with only about 3% of the daily recommended amount. Nutritional yeast grown on a molasses medium is another vegan source of vitamin B12, but not all nutritional yeasts are rich in B12, so check labels for details. Daily recommended intakes for adults are 2.4 mcg and higher if pregnant or nursing.

- **Vitamin C:** Citrus, strawberries, papaya, pineapple, kiwi, cantaloupe, raspberries, bell peppers, broccoli, Brussels sprouts, dark leafy greens, and sweet potato are rich sources of vitamin C.

- **Vitamin E (mixed tocopherols)**: Seeds (especially sunflower seeds), almonds, peanuts, and hazelnuts are rich sources of alpha-tocopherol, and many vegetable oils (e.g., olive oil and canola oil) also contain alpha-tocopherol. Other sources include tomato, avocado, spinach, asparagus, Swiss chard, dark leafy greens, and broccoli.

- **Iron:** Meat, poultry, and fish are some sources. Plant sources include legumes, beans, grains, nuts, seeds, dark leafy greens, prunes, cumin, and raisins. Absorption is increased when consumed with vitamin C.

- **Magnesium**: An essential mineral required for more than 300 biochemical reactions in the body, magnesium is found in a variety of foods including green leafy vegetables, unrefined grains (whole grains), nuts, seeds, and legumes (peas and beans).
- **Selenium**: Sources include fish and shellfish, meat, poultry, cremini mushrooms, shiitake mushrooms, Brazil nuts, some cruciferous vegetables, grains, brown rice, and sunflower seeds.
- **Zinc:** Shellfish, beef, lamb, and turkey are rich sources of zinc. Nuts, seeds, legumes, spinach, asparagus, oats, and yogurt are also good plant sources of zinc.
- **Copper:** This essential trace mineral is found in sesame seeds, cashews, soybeans, shiitake and cremini mushrooms, leafy greens (turnip greens, spinach, Swiss chard, kale, and mustard greens), asparagus, summer squash, legumes, whole grains, nuts, and seeds.
- **Sulfur:** Sulfur compounds are found throughout the body and are needed for metabolism of drugs, steroids, and xenobiotics. They are found in foods such as cruciferous vegetables (broccoli, Brussels sprouts, cauliflower, watercress, cabbage) and allium vegetables (garlic, onions, leeks). Sulfur-containing amino acids are found in animal and cereal proteins.
- **Spices:** Rosemary, basil, turmeric, black pepper, cumin, poppy seeds, and ginger are among culinary herbs and spices that support liver function and can be added into your cooking.
- **Herbs**: Herbs such as milk thistle and dandelion root can protect the liver. These may be consumed as teas or taken in supplement form.

Avoid Liver Stressors

It is best to avoid stressing your liver by moderating your intake of alcohol and minimizing other insults. Current recommendations are to limit daily intake to no more than one alcoholic beverage for women and two for men. Keep your healthcare provider or pharmacist aware of all medications and supplements you take so that they can alert you to possible interactions that could strain your liver function. In addition, limit intake of sugar and simple carbohydrates that reduce the liver's ability to clear chemicals and are associated with diabetes and fatty liver disease. There are many ways to adjust carbohydrate intake to individualize your diet, but in general no more than 30 percent of the calories you consume should come from carbohydrates. The American Heart Association recommends limiting the amount of added sugars to 150 calories per day (about 9 teaspoons) for men and 100 calories per day (about 6 teaspoons) for women.

Consider supplementing with additional detoxification supporting nutrients such as:

- N-acetylcysteine (NAC): 200–500 mg one to three times daily.
- Liposomal glutathione: 250–500 mg two to three times daily.
- Alpha-lipoic acid: 100 mg daily.

11. Drink Green Tea

"Drinking a daily cup of tea will surely starve the apothecary.
- Chinese Proverb

Over the years, there have been many research studies that overwhelmingly support the positive health effects of drinking green tea. Tea (from the plant *Camellia sinensis*) contains polyphenols including epigallocatechin gallate (EGCG), one of the most potent antioxidants. EGCG consumption is associated with reduced incidence of many types of cancer. Green tea helps the body release fat from storage, supports the liver to clean toxins from the blood, and helps fat-soluble toxins leave the body via stool. Drinking green tea protects the heart, benefits mental functioning, and increases levels of normal healthy intestinal bacteria while decreasing levels of disease-causing bacteria. So it's time to pour yourself a cup of tea!

For optimal benefit, drink four to six cups of caffeinated or decaffeinated green tea per day. When choosing a green tea, the tea leaves should be a dark, rich green and have a fresh fragrance. If you choose decaffeinated green tea, find out how the tea was processed to remove the caffeine. Avoid teas that use ethyl acetate to remove the caffeine as it also removes most of the beneficial polyphenols. A different method, called "effervescence," uses water and carbon dioxide, retaining 95 percent of the polyphenols. If you can't get used to the taste of green tea, try white tea, jasmine green tea, matcha tea, or another variety of green tea (there are many). Black tea and oolong tea come from the same plant and have some health benefits, but these tea leaves have been oxidized which reduces the potential antioxidant benefit. Adding citrus juice can significantly boost the bioavailability (the amount of substance that is available to your body) of beneficial compounds. Dairy (such as cream or milk) was formerly suspected to reduce anti-oxidant availability in tea, but further studies show conflicting results. If you just aren't into drinking tea, you may consider taking green tea extracts or EGCG supplements.

But What About My Coffee?

Many studies have shown some health benefits from drinking coffee, and it can be an excellent source of antioxidants. Some people are sensitive to caffeine or the coffee itself, however. This sensitivity may lead people to naturally regulate their coffee intake and may be explained by genetic variations identified by Harvard scientists in 2014. Because of this genetic variation, certain people may be more likely to benefit from increasing or decreasing coffee consumption for optimal health. My take is that if you drink coffee and feel fine, then it's probably fine for you, but choose organic varieties to avoid exposure to pesticides and herbicides and be mindful of what you add to it.

Drinking coffee can become an addictive habit and is sometimes accompanied by other bad habits (the cream and sugar in the coffee or the sweet pastry that goes along with it); it's important to pay attention to how we consume coffee. In addition, when we're stimulated by caffeine, we may not look to foods to provide us with energy and may lack a well-rounded diet. I know that this was the case for me for many years when I was fueled most of the day by coffee and Diet Pepsi and little else of nutritional value.

Prior to starting a detoxification program, it's best to come off of caffeine (of all types) to allow the liver to work optimally and help you get the best results. Remember that the liver is also the primary processor for caffeine, too. Gradually reduce your daily caffeine intake over the course of two to three weeks to avoid symptoms of caffeine withdrawal such as headaches and lethargy. Caffeine has a long half-life (ten to twelve hours), so the cup of coffee that you drink at 8 a.m. is still circulating in your body at half its level at 8 p.m. If you feel poorly while reducing your coffee intake, make sure you are drinking at least six to eight glasses of water and take 1,000 mg buffered vitamin C with breakfast and dinner.

Take a Time-out for Tea:
- **Aim for four to six cups of green tea daily.**
- **If drinking decaffeinated green tea, choose one that uses the effervescence method that retains most of the beneficial polyphenols.**
- **Other varieties to try include white tea, jasmine green tea, or matcha.**

- **Make sure your tea is pesticide-free. Choose USDA Certified Organic brands. Beware of tea grown in China or India. See Resources for recommendations.**
- **Consider green tea extracts or EGCG supplements if you do not enjoy drinking tea.**
- **Other herbal teas or tisanes have different properties and may have other benefits.**

12. Figure Out Your Food Sensitivities

I can't tell you how many patients I have had whose symptoms were unknowingly caused by the foods that they were eating. And in many cases, the foods that were the culprits were the foods that they craved the most! Unlike food allergies, which are caused by immunoglobulin E (IgE) antibody reactions and lead to rashes, hives, and other symptoms including anaphylaxis, food sensitivities can show up as a range of symptoms from brain fog to autoimmune issues to weight gain. When these foods are identified and removed from the diet, many symptoms disappear and the body can heal.

Blood lab analysis for food sensitivity testing is still controversial but can be helpful in certain cases. For some, testing can be a convincing factor to help you realize what needs to be done to move forward for health. It can be hard to hear that you have to break up with bread, for instance. But, for those truly affected by an immune reaction to wheat, seeing definitive lab results may help promote acceptance and adherence to new dietary limitations. In addition, your loved ones may be more supportive of dietary restrictions when there is lab evidence of a problem.

For many, an elimination diet may be the best way to see if you're sensitive to certain foods. To do this, you remove foods that may be triggering symptoms from your diet for one to several weeks. Then, after the elimination period, those foods may be introduced back into your diet to see if they cause a reaction. The Basic Elimination Diet Guide at the end of this book provides details on the process. In my experience this can be a challenging process requiring active support, so in the future I will have a coaching network to help guide you through this process. For starters, I recommend eliminating the top foods that tend to be most reactive for people including wheat and other gluten grains, soy, dairy, eggs, corn, peanuts, and artificial sweeteners, flavorings, and colors. After an elimination period, you will test yourself on these foods by reintroducing them into your diet one at a time over the course of several days to see if you notice a difference in how you feel when that food is brought back. Delicious recipes and tips are provided on how to make this as easy as possible. If you identify a food sensitivity, it is best to remove that food from your diet for at least several months. After a time of desensitization and healing you may try to bring eliminated foods back into your life, but the real litmus test of whether or not you should eat a food is ultimately how you feel. Becoming aware of the effects that the things you consume have on your body and mind is essential to improving your health.

Figuring Out Food Sensitivities

- **Try an elimination diet to determine if you are sensitive to certain foods. See <u>Appendix A</u> for more details.**
- **Consider food sensitivity testing if you are unsure or are overwhelmed by the thought of an elimination diet.**
- **Work with a health practitioner or health coach experienced in food sensitivities and elimination diets if you need support.**

13. Forget That Nonstick Pan and Use Some Elbow Grease

Nonstick pans are one of those miracle timesavers that just might be too good to be true. A while back, warning labels had to be put on nonstick cookware that was treated with Teflon (polytetrafluoroethylene [PTFE] and PFOA [C8]) that cautioned you that it could kill your pet bird. Have you heard the story about the canary in the coal mine? In the old days, canaries were sent down to work with coal miners, and if they died, workers knew there was dangerous gas present and they had to get out of the shaft. Well, if the fumes from the non-stick coating are killing your bird, what are they doing to you? People have been known to be affected by polymer fume fever, which causes a flu-like illness.

In 2006, an EPA Science Advisory board found that PFOA is likely to be carcinogenic in humans and companies that used PFOA were supposed to eliminate it from emissions and product contents by the end of 2015. However, nonstick pans continue to be manufactured and the composition of and safety information on new formulations for these surfaces are difficult to find. Many of these are still in the same family of perfluorinated chemicals or PFCs and are believed to have the same harmful health effects and environmental persistence (see Action Step 5 for more information). To avoid exposure, switch out your nonstick cookware for the following safer options.

Safe Cookware Options to Use:

- **Cast Iron:** Although heavy, these last a lifetime and have the added benefit of boosting your food with iron. Avoid cooking tomato products in cast iron as the acid interacts with the pH of the pan and changes the flavor of the food. Cast iron can be used in the oven or on the stovetop. Keep it seasoned with oil to keep foods from sticking.
- **Porcelain-Enameled Cast Iron:** The enamel surface is easy to cook with and clean (dishwasher-safe), and there is no need to season the cookware. The biggest downside is the cost.
- **Ceramic:** Although breakable, ceramic cookware is great because it doesn't leach anything into food; just make

sure it's lead-free, and don't use anything that is cracked or chipping. You can use steel wool or scrubbing pads without scraping the surface. Some manufacturers are now making cookware that is also coated with ceramic.

- **Glass and Stoneware:** These can be great for baking, but generally can't be used on the stovetop. Stovetop cookware is available in a combination glass-ceramic material.
- **Stainless Steel:** This is made from a combination of metals and quality can differ. Nonmagnetic stainless steel has a very high nickel content which can be allergenic. Use a magnet to test your pans. If it sticks, you have the safer type of pan.
- **Thermolon:** A newer nonstick product that is developed from minerals and supposedly won't break down below temperatures of 450° C (842° F).

Avoid aluminum cookware, which may leach the toxic metal into your food, especially if cooking acidic foods. Consuming large amounts of aluminum may be toxic to the nervous system and has been associated with dementia. Anodized aluminum has been electrochemically altered to make it more stable, but if the surface has been scratched there's a possibility of aluminum leaching into some foods. If using anodized aluminum cookware, check before use for scratches that could potentially cause harm.

Other Tips:
- **Clean surfaces (other than the nonstick variety) using the nontoxic cleaning tips in Action Step 30.**
- **Never preheat nonstick cookware at high heat or put nonstick cookware in an oven hotter than 500° F. Heat at the lowest temperature possible to cook your food safely**
- **Refrain from using the self-cleaning function of your oven as the high temperatures used for this function can release the same fumes as nonstick cookware.**

- **Use an exhaust fan over the stove.**
- **Keep pet birds out of the kitchen.**
- **Replace your cookware as they scratch, peel, and wear out.**

14. Don't Eat or Drink Plastic

Plastic has been an amazing and versatile wonder-material, being used for a variety of things from toothpicks to aircraft. Plastic is convenient, durable, and versatile. But the durability that was once marveled at may be one of the problems as plastics have increasingly invaded our planet, from the products we use to the landfills and oceans and ending up in our tap water. In the United States, we go through about 1,500 plastic water bottles every second! While plastic food containers, bags, and wraps are convenient, one of the main ways we can get plastic chemicals in our bodies is through our food and beverages. Plastics are known to be disrupters of the hormonal system and have been linked to premature sexual development in girls and testicular problems in boys. Exposure to some types of plastic may also increase the risk of cancer.

It is important to never heat food in a plastic container. When a plastic container is labeled "microwave safe," that just means it won't melt during microwaving. Microwave-safe plastics can still leach out and contaminate the food with plastic during microwaving. Food in direct contact with plastic is the most affected, but food that isn't even in contact with the plastic can also become contaminated. If using a microwave, use glass or ceramic containers that are microwave safe. Plastic water bottles left in your hot car or even exposed to heat during shipping can leach chemicals into the water as well, so try to avoid this.

To-go containers can also be a source of toxic chemicals that we end up consuming. Hot foods and beverages can cause leaching of styrene from polystyrene (Styrofoam) cups and food containers. Fast food and greasy takeout food often come in wrappers lined with perfluorocarbons (also known as PFCs), including PFOA, which get into your food. Restaurants and food distributors can opt for different containers and packaging—some of which may even be compostable—and we should all request that they make a switch (see Action Step 5).

It's not just heating that causes contamination. Substances added to plastics to make them soft or pliable, called plasticizers, can contaminate food through simple contact. Plasticizers were found to be high in meat, poultry, fish, and cheese that were packaged in plastic wrapping. Higher levels of plasticizer contamination are found in foods with higher fat content and those wrapped in plastic for a longer period of time. If you can, opt for wraps made from butcher paper, wax paper, or Bee's Wrap, and store food in non-plastic containers once you get it home.

Styrofoam: Bad for Human Health and the Environment

Polystyrene (aka Styrofoam) is one of the most common forms of plastic. Used in a variety of food and beverage containers and packing materials, polystyrene is incredibly durable and is estimated to take at least 500 years to decompose. But despite its low cost and widespread use, over 100 US and Canadian cities, as well as some European and Asian cities, have banned polystyrene food containers and packaging as a result of the negative impacts to humans and the environment. Let's explore why.

Human Health Impact

Polystyrene products contain the toxic substances styrene and benzene, suspected carcinogens and neurotoxins that are known to be hazardous to humans. An estrogenic substance has also been found to be released from polystyrene. Polystyrene food containers can leach out styrene when they come into contact with warm foods and liquids, oily foods, acidic foods (such as citrus fruits), foods that contain vitamin A (such as carrots), and alcohol, causing human contamination and posing a health risk to people.

Effect on Global Warming

According to a 1986 EPA report on solid waste, polystyrene manufacturing was the fifth-largest creator of hazardous waste in the United States. Polystyrene products are made with petroleum, a non-sustainable and heavily polluting resource. If burned, polystyrene releases hazardous carbon monoxide and styrene monomers into the environment. Aside from pollution, environmental impacts of the manufacturing process as well as the use and disposal of polystyrene products include energy consumption, ozone depletion, and greenhouse gas effects.

Water Pollution

People litter polystyrene foam more than any other waste product. Because of its lightweight and buoyant nature, polystyrene is easily blown from disposal sites even when disposed of properly and travels easily through gutters and storm drains, eventually reaching the ocean. Plastic from urban runoff is the largest source of marine debris worldwide, and water pollution negatively affects tourism and quality of life. In addition, polystyrene breaks down into smaller non-biodegradable pieces that are ingested by marine life and other wildlife, thus harming or killing them. It's estimated that polystyrene makes up 60 to 80 percent of marine litter, according to a 2008 review in *Environmental Research*. And because these substances never degrade, microplastics are now found to contaminate 83 percent of the world's tap water. As a result of the impacts on marine pollution and adverse effects to marine wildlife, several coastal cities across the United

States have banned the use of polystyrene food packaging altogether.

Can Polystyrene be Recycled?

While polystyrene may be processed and made into new products like packing materials, they cannot be made into food containers, therefore necessitating the use of resources and hazardous waste creation to continue to provide new food containers. In addition, food containers often cannot be recycled because they have been contaminated with food.

The short-term cost of polystyrene may be low, but the long-term damage is enormous. Polystyrene foam does not decompose and will continue to accumulate in the environment including our food and water until it is banned. This toxin has no place in our bodies, schools, restaurants or homes.

What can we do?
- Be aware of the harmful effects of using polystyrene products and inform others.
- Use reusable cups or more eco-friendly cups instead of polystyrene cups.
- When shopping for groceries, select items that are unwrapped or wrapped in non-polystyrene materials.
- Ask restaurants and food suppliers to use a more environmentally friendly form of food packaging such as those made from post-consumer recycled paper and corn-plastics.

Bisphenol A (BPA), a component of polycarbonate plastic (recycling number 7), is used in drinking bottles, food containers, dental fillings, medical tubing, and the lining of metal food and beverage cans. Scientific evidence shows that BPA acts as a hormone disruptor, contributes to obesity and insulin resistance, and may be linked to cancer, so many manufacturers are now producing BPA-free items. Unfortunately, "BPA-free" products often use Bisphenol S (BPS) and Bisphenol F (BPF), which are known to have similar hormonal effects and should also be avoided. Worse yet, some of the manufacturers are using PVC as a replacement, which is made from carcinogenic vinyl chloride and is known to leach from plastic bottles. Therefore, be mindful of what your food packaging is made of. See the Resources section for some brands that have made an effort to provide nontoxic food packaging.

Plastics are everywhere and they are here to stay—literally. Since they were built to last, they do not biodegrade but rather accumulate in the environment and in us.

The Great Pacific Garbage Patch

Since plastics are not biodegradable, trash from North America, Asia, and activities in the Pacific Ocean have migrated to form the Great Pacific Garbage Patch. No one knows how much debris makes up the Great Pacific Garbage Patch, as it is too large to trawl and much of it is below the surface, but scientists have collected up to 750,000 bits of microplastics in a single square kilometer in this area. Most of this debris comes from plastic bags, bottle caps, plastic water bottles, and polystyrene cups, and its contaminating water and threatening marine life.

Plastic disrupts the marine food web and directly endangers sea life. The debris blocks sunlight from reaching plankton and algae, reducing these food sources for fish and turtles. As their populations diminish, there is less food, in turn, for larger marine life such as tuna, sharks, and whales. In addition, wildlife end up consuming this trash as food, leading to their death from starvation or ruptured organs. Loggerhead sea turtles mistake plastic bags for their favorite food—jellyfish. Albatrosses mistake plastic resin pellets for fish eggs and feed them to their chicks. Seals and other marine mammals are also at risk as they can become entangled in discarded plastic fishing nets and drown.

Plastics can affect marine life by leaching pollutants like BPA out into the environment as they break down. Recent studies have shown that microplastics now contaminate water systems and bottled waters worldwide. Scientists believe that most of the tiny fibers are from clothes, upholstery, and carpets, including particles released in the washing and drying process. Each washing machine cycle potentially releases more than 700,000 microscopic plastic particles. These microplastics can absorb harmful pollutants linked to cancer and other illnesses, such as PCBs, which are then consumed by fish, farm animals, and humans.

Plastics by the Numbers
Look for the number stamped in the middle of the triangular recycling symbol (the Resin Identification Code [RIC]) to help determine what type of plastic a product is made of.

Less toxic plastics:
1 - **Polyethylene Terephthalate (PET or PETE)**: single-use bottles and containers; may release antimony; recyclable
2 - **High-Density Polyethylene (HDPE)**: used for milk jugs, cereal bags, shampoo bottles, toys, etc.; may release estrogenic chemicals; recyclable
4 - **Low-Density Polyethylene (LDPE)**: juice and milk cartons, plastic wrap, grocery and garbage bags; recyclable
5 - **Polypropylene (PP)**: syrup, ice cream and yogurt containers, drinking straws, salad bar containers, diapers, plastic cups, baby bottles, microwavable plastic containers and lids; recyclable.

7 – "Other" Plastics: look for newer PLA (polymer polylactide), which is typically made from corn or sugarcane and is not recyclable but may be compostable. No health risks have yet been identified for PLA which does not contain BPA. Since #7 is a catch-all number, make sure it says "PLA."

More toxic plastics:

3 – Polyvinyl Chloride (PVC): cling wrap, some food containers, shower curtains, bibs, etc. Vinyl chloride is a known carcinogen. PVC also includes phthalates, which interfere with hormone development. The manufacture of PVC creates PCBs and dioxin, a potent carcinogen that contaminates humans, animals, and the environment.

6 – Extruded Polystyrene (PS): commonly known as Styrofoam. Leaches styrene, a carcinogen and neurotoxin. Worse when heated, such as drinking coffee from a polystyrene cup. Also used in egg cartons, disposable cutlery, packing materials, and CD and DVD cases.

7 – "Other" Plastics: often times refers to polycarbonate (PC). Used for baby bottles, watercooler jugs, and epoxy linings of tin cans. PC is composed of BPA, which is linked to cancer and obesity, or BPS, which has been shown to have similar endocrine effects.

To Reduce the Effects of Toxic Plastics:

- Store food and beverages in reusable glass and 100% stainless-steel containers. Use glass or stainless-steel water bottles without plastic linings.
- Don't leave plastic water bottles in your hot car.
- Don't microwave plastics or fill them with hot liquids or foods. If you must store food in plastic, allow the food to cool before putting it in the container.
- Only put plastics in the freezer if they have a freezer-safe label. Freezer temperatures can cause plastics to degrade, increasing leaching into food when thawed.

- **Look for nontoxic reusable lunch boxes and bags made without vinyl or lead.**
- **Wash plastic food containers by hand or on the top shelf of the dishwasher, where the water is cooler.**
- **Avoid using old, scratched plastic water bottles or food containers.**
- **Minimize single-use plastic bags, containers, and other items that are intended for single-use but last a lifetime. Bring reusable shopping bags and containers with you. If the situation permits, pass on the coffee or soda cup lid and plastic straws.**
- **Instead of plastic wrap, use wraps made from butcher paper, wax paper, or Bee's Wrap.**
- **Suggest to restaurants and food service facilities that they use compostable or recyclable food containers.**
- **Recycle according to your local waste management company directions.**
- **If you see plastic litter, dispose of it properly so that it does not end up harming wildlife and contaminating water.**

15. Eat the Six Tastes

According to Ayurveda, we experience six main tastes of food: sweet, sour, salty, pungent, bitter, and astringent. When we experience all of these tastes in a balanced manner, we obtain a complete array of nutrients as well as a complete sensory experience that relays information to our brain, creating harmony in mind and body.

Sweet is not just cookies and candies. It is the taste of nourishment and builds tissues. We get the sweet taste from proteins, fats, and carbohydrates found in grains, nuts, seeds, oils, dairy, sweet fruits, starchy vegetables, animal products, and typically sweet things such as sugar and honey. The key is to have balance and to make sure that the information that is being relayed by your food—the nutrient value—is high quality. There is a huge difference in the information provided by 100 calories worth of a chemical-laden Twinkie versus 100 calories worth of a phytonutrient-rich sweet potato. Which do you think is going to send a message of health to your DNA and ultimately to your body?

Sour promotes appetite and digestion, and we experience the sour taste from the acids contained in the foods. This taste is in citrus fruits, berries, tomatoes, sour fruits, and foods which have been fermented, such as yogurt, cheese, vinegar, pickled foods, kimchi, kombucha, and alcohol. The positive impact that fermented foods have on our gut microbiome has recently increased their popularity. The key here is to get the right amount. Too much of the sour taste can exacerbate heartburn, especially in those who are prone to this condition. As a side note, while acid-blockers and proton-pump inhibitors are useful in the repair and prevention of mucosal injury to the upper gastrointestinal tract, prolonged use of them has been associated with vitamin and mineral deficiencies, alteration in gut flora, and more serious health conditions. If you have been taking daily medication to reduce acid, talk to your healthcare provider about the possibility of gradually weaning off of them.

The **salty** taste also promotes digestion, and while we commonly think of salt as sodium chloride, other mineral salts such as calcium, magnesium, and potassium are important and necessary for our body processes. We get the salty taste from table salt, sea salt, seafood, sea vegetables, meats, condiments, and sauces. Again, moderation is key. And if you are among the 25 percent of the population that is sensitive to salt, you should eat a low-sodium diet (usually less than 2,000 mg of sodium per day) to lower the risks of high blood pressure, stroke, heart attack, and kidney disease.

The standard American diet is chock full of the sweet, sour, and salty tastes just described but is usually lacking in the pungent, bitter, and astringent tastes which are naturally built in to many cuisines from around the world. If you find that you're missing these tastes, start to incorporate them with the foods described below to provide balance as well as a variety of beneficial nutrients.

Pungent foods are naturally detoxifying and stimulate digestion. Just think of the warmth that comes from eating herbs and spices like pepper, cayenne, chilies, ginger, garlic, onions, leeks, radish, horseradish, mustard, basil, thyme, cloves, and cinnamon. Not only are these foods heating to our body, possibly making our eyes water and our noses run and causing us to flush or even break a sweat (all detoxifying actions), but the phytochemicals (plant-based natural chemical compounds) in some of these herbs and spices actually support all three phases of detoxification. If some of these are too spicy for you, choose cooler herbs and spices that also support the liver and can have other beneficial health effects such as rosemary, cilantro, coriander, and turmeric. Go ahead and spice it up!

Bitter foods are often the least palatable but can be among the most anti-inflammatory and detoxifying foods for us. Many medicinal plants fall under the bitter category and this taste, when too much, can cause us to want to spit it out. This is to protect us naturally from consuming toxic plants which also often contain bitter compounds. In many cases, the dose makes the poison: a little bit is good for you, but excess can lead to danger. When we consume a bitter taste, our digestive tract is stimulated to move along, pushing the contents out of our system more quickly as a further protection from potentially poisonous plants. Because of this effect, digestive bitters are often given to help facilitate digestion especially in those with a sluggish system. Foods in this category include leafy greens, green and yellow squash, broccoli, and other cruciferous vegetables. The phytochemicals in these plants also support liver detoxification systems.

The last taste described in Ayurveda is more of a sensation, as there are no receptors for this taste on the tongue. When we eat **astringent** foods, they act to pull water. Think of what your mouth and tongue feel like if you drink a cup of black tea that has been steeping too long or if you drink a glass of straight unsweetened cranberry juice or bite into an unripe, green banana. That puckering sensation comes from the astringent properties of the polyphenols found in dark-pigmented fruits, tea, and legumes. These foods also have high fiber content and the polyphenols give these superfoods disease-fighting power. The compacting action of astringent foods helps to balance over-accumulation of fluids which can be helpful for symptoms such as chronic sinus drainage, loose stool, and edema.

While each of these tastes is necessary for optimal health, the balance of how much to eat of each type depends on a person's constitution, known as *dosha* in Ayurveda. Determining your *dosha* and learning to balance your mind-body physiology can be complex, and I incorporate this valuable tool in my clinical practice and coaching programs. See the Resources section for Chapter 4 to find out more about Ayurveda. To begin with, start by going beyond the tastes of sweet, sour, and salty and experience the pungent, bitter, and astringent tastes every day and eventually in every meal. As you progress, you can then learn to eat right for your *dosha* which can be an important tool in optimizing your mind-body function. Many of my patients have had profound shifts in their health and well-being just by making a few simple changes to balance their *doshas*, including eliminating heartburn, chronic sinusitis, irritable bowel symptoms, and constipation.

16. Optimize Digestion with Mindful Eating

It's so easy to eat mindlessly—grabbing a handful of candy left out on the office counter, mowing through an entire bag of chips while watching TV, eating food just because it is there and not necessarily because it is healthy and nourishing for us at that time. The key is to shift from consuming foods "just because" to choosing foods that make you feel vital, energetic, and joyful. This takes attention and intention. Here are some simple tips to maximize your eating enjoyment.

Before you eat, first sit down, allowing the blood to circulate to your digestive tract. Take a good look at your food. Does it include all of the six tastes (see Action Step 15)? Does it include a rainbow of colors (see Action Step 1)? Consider where the food came from, beginning with the seed and the soil, the energy that it harnessed from the sun, the growth of the plant, and, if it's an animal product, also consider the conditions that it was raised in, its food sources, and its environment. Consider who looked after this food while it was being formed, who harvested it. How did it travel to you, and what, if any, processing was involved? And finally, who prepared the meal, and was it prepared and served out of love? Give gratitude for the food that you are about to consume that will ultimately be incorporated into your body.

Notice your mental and emotional state. If you are distracted, upset, or stressed, your food will be metabolized differently, going down a pathway that leads to inflammation and potentially creating toxicity. Distracted or emotional eating can also lead you to consume more food than you normally would. Are you able to enjoy the sensory experience of your food, or are you multi-tasking—watching TV, reading, working, texting? And finally, consider who you are eating with. Are you alone or with someone whose company you enjoy or perhaps don't enjoy? All of these factors play a role in how much you eat as well as how you will digest and metabolize your food.

It is important to eat only when you are hungry and stop before you are too full. Think of your appetite as a scale of zero to ten: zero being completely empty and ravenous and ten being post-Thanksgiving feast where you feel the need to unbutton your pants. Eat when you feel truly hungry at about a level two—the last meal has been digested and your stomach is ready to accept new fuel. Prevent yourself from getting to a zero where your blood sugar has dipped so low that you can barely function. Waiting this long makes it more likely that you will eat whatever is easily available to you, which may not be the healthiest choice. When famished we also tend to eat quickly, leading to overeating. Eat at a moderate pace, making sure to chew your foods well, since digestion begins in the mouth with chewing and the release of salivary enzymes. It takes twenty minutes for your brain to register that food is in your stomach, so make sure you are taking enough time to eat and digest your meal. Oftentimes we mistake thirst for hunger, so also make sure you are well-hydrated between meals.

We need to be mindful of portion sizes on our plates. Many Americans have become accustomed to huge plates that are filled to the rim, while the size of our stomach is about the size of our fist. The stomach does expand to accommodate the volume of food consumed, but the ability to digest is reduced when we overeat. We're also more likely to accumulate toxic buildup (known as *ama* in Ayurveda) and experience discomfort, bloating, and heartburn if we overeat. If you're accustomed to having an overflowing plate, reduce your portion size gradually and you'll soon realize how great you can feel from not overindulging. One helpful trick is to use smaller plates or only use the interior part of the plate instead of filling it to the outer edges. Our plate sizes have drastically increased over the last eighty or so years; a contractor friend of mine who rehabs older homes from the 1920s to 1950s often has to replace kitchen cabinets because our modern-day plates are just too big! As you consume your food, focus on its taste, aroma, and texture: studies have found that simply paying mindful attention to one's food in this way leads to less intake.

To optimize your digestive capacity, eat the largest meal of the day mid-day when your digestive fire (*agni*) is at its strongest. Metabolism slows during the latter part of the day, so dinner should be light and easily digestible in contrast to our typical large Western evening meal. If we overeat in the evening, it can lead to digestive as well as sleep difficulties. About six hours after we consume carbohydrates, our body secretes the hormone leptin, which signals satiety to the brain and keeps hunger at bay during the night. Avoid late-night snacking, as fasting overnight turns on genes that break down fat and cholesterol. We must fast for five or six hours for this switch to turn on, and then we must continue fasting to metabolize the calories we have accumulated during the day. In the morning, adrenaline and cortisol are at their peak making it an ideal time to break the fast.

Mindful Eating Tips:
- **Sit down to eat.**
- **Mindfully consider the tastes and origins of your food, and practice gratitude.**
- **Avoid eating when distracted, upset, or acutely stressed.**
- **Eat only when hungry and stop before you are too full.**
- **Adjust your portion size to the amount appropriate for your body size and metabolism.**
- **Eat the largest meal at mid-day when your digestive ability is strongest. Eat smaller, easily digestible meals in the evening when digestion tends to be weaker.**
- **Fast at least six hours overnight.**

Chapter 6.
What Goes On: Skin, Body, and Clothing

"If you wouldn't put it in your body, why would you put it on your body?"

- Horst Rechelbacher, founder of Aveda

While food provides the basic building blocks, our bodies are made from an interaction between our DNA (which provides the basic code) and the environment (which modulates which codes get to be played out). It turns out that we cannot blame our genes completely for the current state of our health except in rare cases. As science has shown, there are many factors to determine the state of our health including our lifestyle, the balance of microorganisms living in and on our body, and the substances we come into contact with in our personal environment.

Scientists have learned a tremendous amount in the last decade about the microbes that live with us, called our microbiome. Beneficial microbes help with digestion, metabolism, production and absorption of nutrients, immune function, and even our mood. We are going from an era when bacteria were the targeted enemy to encouraging their proper balance through food and nutrients. There is still so much to learn, but there is no doubt about the huge impact these little organisms have on our health.

Another area where we can make a big impact is by paying attention to what goes on our biggest organ—our skin. Next to optimizing what we eat, noticing what we put on our skin is another area where we can greatly reduce our toxic load. From personal care products to clothing, we come into contact with hundreds of ingredients each day that are not fully regulated for safety and can be absorbed into our body through our skin. What is the point of spending time and energy to eat organic, wholesome foods if you are still slathering neurotoxins and endocrine disruptors on your body? In several sections of this chapter, I will tell you what to look for and how to detox this area of your life.

Certain practices can also enhance detoxification through a balanced daily routine. Releasing toxins through sweat, breathing exercises, and Ayurvedic cleansing techniques can help you on your journey to health and wellness. As you begin to incorporate these practices regularly, you will strengthen your vitality and increase your body's natural capacity for healing.

17. Your Genes Are Not Your Destiny

In 2003, the Human Genome Project completed the enormous task of mapping the three billion chemical base pairs that contain all the information needed for human life and was thought to also contain vital information to prevent or cure disease. But it turns out that figuring out our genetic blueprint is only part of the story. In fact, only 5 percent of genes have a fixed effect, meaning 95 percent of our genes are actually flexible in their expression—they can be turned on or off in response to our environment and everything that we think or do. Evolutionarily, this is a great advantage, allowing our bodies to adapt to changing environments and circumstances, to turn on growth and repair mechanisms when needed and turn them off when the job is finished. But we can run into problems when genes regulating inflammation are turned on and then are not turned back off or when repair genes should be turned on but aren't.

Looking at gene expression and what influences it is as important as finding out what genes we were born with. Whether or not a gene is expressed is greatly impacted by your lifestyle. What you eat, how much physical activity you do, your level of stress, exposure to environmental toxins—these all serve to communicate to your genome, determining how your body will respond. In the field of functional medicine there is a saying, "The genes load the gun, but the environment and lifestyle pulls the trigger." This helps to account for studies of identical twins who, despite being born with the same genetic makeup, can have drastically different health outcomes—who we become is shaped by our life experiences interacting with our genome.

For the majority of people who do not have a gene for some rare form of disease, the gene variants that we inherit merely determine a susceptibility for illness or wellness and are not a guarantee of actually suffering from disease. So the question should go beyond "Do I have this gene?" to "Do I have a lifestyle that leads to helpful or harmful genetic activity?" Every cell is eavesdropping on what you think, say, and do, so it is wise to do your best to optimize your gene activity by optimizing the message that your genes receive. In this way, you are able to mitigate the effects of certain genetic predispositions.

Our genetic differences are one reason why a one-size-fits-all approach to medical treatment doesn't necessarily work. In medical school, we always discussed cases using a hypothetical 70 kg (150 lb.) male. It was assumed that most everyone would respond to medications in exactly the same way. But we now know that how people respond is highly individualized, and medicine therefore needs to move toward a more personalized approach to treatment. One of the ways that genes vary is in what are called single nucleotide polymorphisms (SNPs). For instance, if you have a SNP (pronounced "snip") in one or more of the liver detox CYP450 enzymes, you might have difficulty metabolizing certain medications leading you to be sensitive to lower doses, have an increased likelihood of side effects, and keep the medication in your system for a longer period of time. Gene testing for some of these SNPs is available and is also becoming less costly, but it still is not widely covered by health insurance. I really don't advocate treating the presence of a SNP due to testing alone, however, as one always must take into account the entire patient picture.

Methylation and detoxification pathways are very commonly affected by SNPs, particularly in patients who become affected by environmental overload. Methylation is a process of adding a methyl group (carbon and three hydrogens) to a compound and is important in hundreds of reactions in the body including detoxification, synthesis of neurotransmitters, formation of enzymes and proteins, protecting our telomeres (protective end-caps on our chromosomes), and metabolism of certain vitamins and amino acids. Beyond the methylation cycle, other processes are also essential to detoxification and metabolism. Presence of SNPs can cause too much or too little of certain biochemicals to be made, resulting in health effects downstream. When I find out a patient has one or more SNPs, I explain that it's like you are trying to get from Los Angeles to San Diego, but some of the freeway on-ramps and off-ramps are closed. That doesn't necessarily mean that you can't get there. It just means you are going to have to take some detours, your trip may take longer, and you will end up using more resources to reach your goal. By determining which enzymes and processes may be affected by the SNPs, you can utilize food, nutrients, and lifestyle to optimize functioning. Even if we cannot reverse a person's SNPs, we can get them functioning and feeling a whole lot better

In addition to lifestyle factors that regulate gene expression to impact our current level of functioning, the effect of environmental and lifestyle influences on gene expression can reach beyond our individual lifetime to affect future generations.

How you live today can be transferred to the well-being of your children, their children, and beyond, through what is known as the epigenome. Epidemiologic studies have shown multigenerational effects after famine, toxic exposures, and psychological stress. In addition, there is also a concept of the social genome whereby our social interactions with others can also affect gene expression.

So what can we do with this information? As I mentioned before, all of our life experiences influence which genes get activated and which ones don't. Thus far, the impact of food has been found to be the most influential and nutrigenomics is the science that studies how food and nutrition affect gene expression. Reducing environmental and psychological stress can also turn our healthy genes on and our disease genes off. A recent study that we conducted at the Chopra Center showed that practicing meditation for just four days affected gene expression even in novice meditators, while more experienced regular meditators showed more robust results, indicating a practice effect. Knowing about our genes and our particular susceptibilities, we can make diet and lifestyle choices that minimize expression of disease genes and maximize expressions of health and longevity genes.

Tips to Optimize Your Gene Expression:

- **Eat a clean and nutrient-rich diet (See Action Steps 1-12).**
- **Reduce your environmental load by reducing exposures and support detoxification processes.**
- **Use stress management techniques regularly. Meditation has been shown to influence gene expression, turning on healthy genes and turning down disease genes.**
- **Consider gene testing to be able to address certain susceptibilities including SNPs that may affect methylation and detoxification.**

- **Consider micronutrient testing to identify nutritional deficiencies that can affect multiple processes in the body including the ability to detoxify.**

18. Nurture Your Inner Garden

Each of us is born with 23,000 genes of our own and no microbes, but after passing through the birth canal, breastfeeding, and being around other people and pets, a baby soon becomes colonized with symbiotic bacteria which we call our microbiome. It is estimated that we harbor 100 trillion gut microbes with at least 1,000 different species whose genes outnumber ours by 150 to 1. While we have become accustomed to think of microbes as bad for us (and that is true for pathogenic microbes such as *Salmonella* and *E. coli*), we evolved with these microbes over the course of human development, and our microbiome actually plays an essential role in digestion, production of nutrients including vitamin B12 and the neurotransmitter serotonin, regulating inflammation, processing of wastes, and immune system function.

Our personal microbiome is affected by many factors: our mother's microbiome, being born vaginally or by cesarean section, exposure to antibiotics, having been breastfed or not, the environment where we were born and where we live, the people and pets that we are exposed to, the foods that we eat, stress level, exposure to environmental toxins, and hormonal changes. These factors have likely contributed to a decrease in biodiversity as well as decreased number of organisms that we see in most people today. Science is just beginning to explore the importance of our microbiome; however, it has become clear that changes in our inner ecology may be at the root of many of our modern health epidemics including food allergies, autoimmune illnesses, digestive disorders, obesity, diabetes, and heart disease. Research is also pointing to the influence of our microbiome on epigenetic regulation.

While beneficial microbes are found in and on many areas of the body, the gut microbiome plays a particularly important role, especially for informing our immune system. The normal state of our gut lining is an intact barrier, preventing transport of large molecules into the bloodstream and allowing chosen digested nutrients to pass through. Bacteria in the small intestine help to protect this barrier, which can be damaged by drugs, toxins, oxidative stress, and disease (celiac, infection, inflammatory bowel disease). If there is a breakdown in this barrier, as happens when a person has "leaky gut," incompletely digested food particles, including large proteins, can pass from the gut to the bloodstream causing an inflammatory and immune response. Because some of these component particles mimic human tissues, this can also create an autoimmune response. In this way, foods that previously were never problematic to a person can become triggers.

Aside from taking in nutrients to use as building blocks for our body, our gut has a major role in interactions with the world around us—training the immune system as well as informing our mood and emotions. When we consider that what we ingest is a major way in which we are exposed to our environment on a daily basis, it makes sense that 60 to 80 percent of our total immune system is in the gastrointestinal tract as Gut-Associated Lymphatic Tissue (GALT). It is also estimated that 80 to 95 percent of the total amount of the neurotransmitter serotonin in our bodies is manufactured in the gut, and gut bacteria manufacture dozens of other neurochemicals as well. So when we say we have a "gut feeling," it is likely due to this powerful link between the brain, the gut, and the microbiome.

If you have developed a leaky gut, repair is necessary to prevent further attacks on your system. Treatment includes removing items from your diet and lifestyle that continue to cause further injury and ensuring a healthy inner environment with adequate nutrients for repair and defense including the amino acid glutamine, prebiotics, and probiotics. However, even if you do not have leaky gut, maintenance of your inner flora is essential to your health.

The first step in supporting your gut microbiome is to make sure that you are providing the right nutrients for beneficial bacteria while decreasing food sources for pathogenic bacteria. Studies have shown that the composition of gut flora can be changed very rapidly and reproducibly in response to dietary changes. Bacteria are able to digest nutrients that humans cannot due to specialized enzymes, and these nutrients are called prebiotics. Although all prebiotics are fiber, not all fiber is prebiotic. Prebiotics occur naturally in foods such as leeks, asparagus, chicory, Jerusalem artichokes, garlic, onions, wheat, oats, and soybeans. Fermentable fiber from these foods feeds certain bacteria that produce beneficial short-chain fatty acids (SCFA) which provide a variety of functions including serving as fuel for our intestinal cells. Butyrate is a particular SCFA which also has anti-inflammatory properties and increases insulin sensitivity. Bacterial species can be so specialized that they digest specific subtypes of fiber differently. For this reason, I recommend eating a variety of vegetables and fruits. Eating a very low-carbohydrate diet, on the other hand, may starve both good and bad gut bacteria.

Fibers that ferment quickly may lead to excessive gas production and bloating, so if that tends to be an issue for you, choose fiber that ferments little and slowly such as the peel of an apple or the stems of broccoli, and stay away from rapidly fermentable fiber such as inulin from onions, asparagus, leek, banana, wheat, and garlic. Each vegetable or fruit will contain several types of fiber and everyone's microbiome is different, so you will have to individualize based on what you tolerate. I prefer that people consume whole foods which naturally contain fiber as well as a host of other phytonutrients rather than take a fiber supplement, but sometimes that is also needed.

What is SIBO?

If you have chronic abdominal bloating, you may have a condition called small intestinal bacterial overgrowth, or SIBO. This is a result of imbalances in gut bacteria that have favored the strains that enjoy fermenting starchy carbs or fermentable oligosaccharides, disaccharides, monosaccharides, and polyols (FODMAPs). By consuming a low-FODMAP diet you will starve out these strains, resulting in decreased symptoms and addressing the underlying cause of the bacterial imbalance in the gut. SIBO is a common cause of Irritable Bowel Syndrome (IBS), and treating the overgrowth can greatly improve IBS symptoms. Symptoms of SIBO include: bloating/abdominal gas; flatulence and belching; abdominal pain, discomfort, or cramps; constipation, diarrhea, or a mixture of the two; heartburn; and nausea. Aside from annoying symptoms, bacterial overgrowth can also impair digestion and absorption and lead to certain nutrient deficiencies and systemic issues. If you suspect that you have SIBO, contact a healthcare provider who may order a breath test to determine if you have it. Medical treatment may be necessary.

Consuming oral probiotics and probiotic-rich foods can also help to support your bacterial flora by introducing more friendly bacteria into your digestive tract. If you have digestive issues or serious health problems, be sure to start slowly, otherwise you could throw yourself into a whole new kind of imbalance. Probiotic-rich foods include fermented foods such as yogurt with active cultures (but watch the sugar content), kefir, sauerkraut, kimchee, kombucha, pickles, other fermented vegetables, natto, miso, tempeh, and raw cheese. Most store-bought yogurt contains a lot of sugar and may only contain a small amount of the beneficial bacteria *Lactobacillus acidophilus*, so be sure to read the label. Look for "live active cultures," since yogurt that is pasteurized after it is made ends up with no beneficial bacteria as they are destroyed in the pasteurization process. Make sure your dairy products have not been produced with antibiotics or hormones. For those sensitive to dairy, there are now coconut yogurts and kefirs on the market.

There are many probiotic supplements available and they come in liquid or capsule form. Many probiotic bacteria, particularly those with live cultures, are naturally sensitive to heat and moisture and should be refrigerated and kept out of humidity. However, freeze-dried probiotics in blister packs have longer shelf lives and may be fine as long as they are not exposed to heat above room temperature. Probiotic yeast (*Saccharomyces boulardii*) and some of the spore-forming bacteria, such as *Bacillus coagulans*, generally do not require refrigeration. Look for a supplement that contains at least both *Lactobacillus* and *Bifidobacterium* families and with at least five to twenty billion live bacteria per dose. Take once or twice daily. Those with IBS or Inflammatory Bowel Disease (IBD) may require higher-dose supplements such as VSL#3, which has 250 billion live bacteria per dose. The best probiotic supplements will use delivery systems that ensure a significantly high percentage of bacteria will reach your intestines alive. Expiration dates on probiotic supplements indicate that the bacteria in the product should be active and potent at the levels indicated on the label until that date. Usually the expiration date is based on formulation and stability testing data, which means a company is paying attention to those matters. Look for reputable brands (see the Resources section for more information); you do get what you pay for.

Because the different strains of probiotic bacteria have slightly different functions and are concentrated in various places along the digestive tract, probiotic supplements that contain multiple strains may be more useful for supporting the general microbiome. I usually recommend products that contain several strains of both *Lactobacillus* and *Bifidobacterium* families: *L. acidophilus*, which supports digestion, nutrient, immune health, and urinary tract and vaginal health in women; *L. fermentum*, which supports digestion and detoxification; *L. rhamnosus*, which can be helpful for traveler's diarrhea and vaginal health in women; *L. plantarum* for digestion and immune health; *B. longum*, which helps maintain gut integrity and process toxins; *B. bifidum*, which supports digestion and nutrient absorption; and *B. infantis*, which supports digestion and can help with occasional bloating and constipation. At times I recommend a specific strain that has been clinically studied for a particular condition. For example, *L. rhamnosus* GR-1 and *L. reuteri* RC-14 are two highly studied probiotic strains for women's health. The letters and numbers that appear after the name is the particular pedigree of the bacteria and, although not necessary for a good product, indicate that the company is using a pure, genetically characterized strain.

Antibiotics

Antibiotics have saved many lives, but killing bad (pathogenic) bacteria can also kill the good flora in our gut, skin, mouth, and vagina that we need to thrive. And unfortunately antibiotics have been used too widely in the medical profession as well as in animal husbandry, creating drug-resistant superbugs and drastically altering our gut microbiome. That's not to say that antibiotics are all bad, and if you have a serious infection they may certainly be necessary. Microbial flora may be restored after the antibiotic is stopped, but when the microbial balance is disrupted it can lead to dysbiosis—an imbalance in the ecology of the gut—creating digestive problems as well as systemic illnesses. Dysbiosis has been linked to asthma, eczema, autoimmune illnesses, Crohn's multiple sclerosis, autism, Alzheimer's rheumatoid arthritis, lupus, obesity, cardiovascular disease, atherosclerosis, cancer, and malnutrition.

Supporting Your Microbiome:

- Eat less sugar, refined carbohydrates, and alcohol.
- Eat more anti-inflammatory foods like vegetables, fruits, whole grains, nuts, seeds, and omega-3 rich foods.
- Eat fermentable fiber from whole fruits, vegetables, and grains.
- Eat probiotic rich foods like yogurt, sauerkraut, kimchee, kombucha, and other fermented vegetables, and take a probiotic supplement.
- Avoid chemically processed foods and GMO foods.
- Use antibiotics wisely and avoid them in your food supply.
- Utilize stress management practices.
- Find out more about your microbial balance with testing. See the Resources section.

19. Beauty is More than Skin Deep – Clean Up Your Personal Care Products

Many personal care products look good on the surface but are actually laden with chemicals that can cause harmful effects, including carcinogens, endocrine disruptors, and allergens. So if you spend a lot of time considering what you put *into* your body but not what you put *on* your body, you are missing a huge source of potential toxicity. Our skin is our largest organ covering about twenty square feet, and a large part of what we put on our skin is absorbed. From moisturizers, perfumes, lipsticks, fingernail polishes, cosmetics, hair care products, toothpastes, and deodorant, the average woman uses 12 products containing 168 unique ingredients every day, while men on average use 6 products daily with 85 unique ingredients.

The National Institute of Occupational Safety and Health (NIOSH) found more than 2,500 chemicals in cosmetics that can cause skin and eye irritations, tumors, reproductive issues, and mutations in animals and possibly humans. Unfortunately, the personal care product industry's self-policing safety panel, the Cosmetic Ingredient Review (CIR) does not require safety testing for its products and more than 80 percent of products have not been tested. As a result, almost any material may be used as a cosmetic ingredient without approval from the FDA. And while the European Union has banned or regulated more than 1,300 ingredients in personal care products, the United States has only banned eleven. In the cosmetics industry, labels like "organic," "natural," "pure," "hypoallergenic," "botanical," "green," "eco," "nontoxic," and "FDA-approved" are unregulated and therefore meaningless, leading to greenwashing claims that make products appear more environmentally friendly and less toxic. Unfortunately, even if a product contains actual organic ingredients, it may be packaged right along with toxic and synthetic chemicals.

What is an Endocrine Disruptor?

The endocrine (hormonal) system is an important and complex system responsible for regulating everything from our mood, to our reproductive processes, to our growth and development, to our sexual function and metabolism. Endocrine disruptors are chemicals that mimic our own hormones and may play a role in reproductive issues such as low sperm count and infertility, metabolic dysregulation, early pubertal development, cancer, and birth defects. These effects can occur at even very small microdoses.

To clean up your personal care products, look for products with fewer chemicals, avoid synthetic fragrances (see Action Step 29), and use fewer products overall, especially on children or while pregnant. If you follow the advice of "If you wouldn't eat it, don't put it on your skin," you will likely be safe. If you are unsure of your product or its ingredients, check the EWG's Skin Deep database, which rates products on their level of potential to cause cancer, allergic reactions, hormonal issues, reproductive problems, and damage to a developing fetus. Choose products that are given a rating of 0 to 2, which is the least toxic range. The EWG's Healthy Living app has the ability to search by product name or use a barcode scanner to conveniently determine if the product scores well or not. While many companies have responded to consumer demand for safer products, some still score all over the map so it is important to look at each product individually.

Ingredients to Avoid:

- fragrance/perfume/parfum
- all "parabens"
- sodium laureth sulfate (SLES). Try to avoid ingredients that start with "PEG" or have an "-eth" in the middle.
- quaternium-15
- DMDM hydantoin
- imidazolidinyl urea
- diazolidinyl urea
- sodium hydroxymethylglycinate
- 2-bromo-2-nitropropane-1,3 diol (Bronopol)
- DBP, DEHP, DEP
- PTFE
- methylchloroisothiazolinone, methylisothiazolinone
- oxybenzone
- triclosan, triclocarban
- triethanolamine (or "TEA")
- FD&C, D&C

Tips to Detox Your Personal Care Products:

- Use fewer products and use them less often.
- Buy products with fewer ingredients.
- Buy fragrance-free products.
- Don't trust advertising hype. Beware of greenwashing.
- Check ingredients with EWG's Skin Deep database.
- Avoid the use of baby/talcum powder, which has been linked to ovarian cancer.
- Beware of "pinkwashing." Some companies market themselves as champions of women's health, putting a pink ribbon on their products and donating a portion of proceeds to breast cancer charities while continuing to put carcinogens and endocrine disruptors in their products.

20. Be Sunscreen Savvy

We have all heard the news that we should use sunscreen to protect ourselves from skin cancer as well as prevent signs of aging, but not all sunscreens are created equal. Each year, the EWG evaluates the ingredients and effectiveness of over 1,500 sunscreens and SPF-rated moisturizers and lip balms, with particular attention to effectiveness as well as skin penetration, effects on the hormonal system, presence in breast milk, issues with child development, allergic skin reactions, potential for inhalation, chemical stability, and other toxicity concerns including carcinogenic and neurotoxic effects. In 2017, the EWG's Guide to Sunscreens found that many brands made inaccurate and misleading claims and advised consumers to be wary of labels with claims of "water-proof," "broad-spectrum protection," "chemical-free," "for babies," "natural," and any SPF over 50. They found that some of the worst products were the more popular brands, so how do you know what is good or not?

Today's sunscreens work either by mineral or chemical filters. The most common sunscreens on the market contain chemical filters that typically include a combination of some of these active ingredients: oxybenzone, avobenzone, octisalate, octocrylene, homosalate, and octinoxate (octylmethoxycinnamate). These chemical sunscreens are absorbed through the skin and enter the bloodstream, circulating through the entire body and potentially causing harm. The chemicals have been detected in the blood, urine, and breast milk up to two days after a single application. Oxybenzone, octinoxate, and homosalate are all hormone disrupters. Avobenzone must be stabilized with another chemical and often causes skin sensitivity. Octocrylene in the presence of UV light (sunlight) can produce free radicals and may harm the environment. In addition, chemical sunscreens such as oxybenzone have been shown to destroy coral reefs at a concentration of sixty-two parts per trillion (the equivalent of a drop of water in an Olympic swimming pool). Coral reefs are important for local economies and also help the global environment through their absorption of carbon dioxide that would otherwise contribute to global warming.

Mineral sunscreens use zinc oxide or titanium dioxide, which form a physical barrier as these minerals "float" on the top of the skin and are not absorbed. While mineral filters are not endocrine disruptors and have not been shown to cause damage to coral reefs, there is caution about the use of nanoparticle formulations, which may absorb into the skin as well as end up contaminating the environment. Some products use both mineral and chemical filters.

In addition to being careful about the active ingredient in sunscreens, avoid products with retinyl palmitate, a form of vitamin A that was found by the EWG to be added to 13 to 18 percent of evaluated products. Studies suggest that retinyl palmitate may speed the development of skin tumors when applied to skin in the presence of sunlight. It may also be listed in products as retinol, retinyl acetate, retinyl linoleate, and retinoic acid. Other ingredients of concern include perfume/

parfum/fragrance (see Action Step 29) and methylisothiazo-linone (MI), a preservative which can cause allergic reactions and may be neurotoxic.

Another aspect to consider is that sunscreen use can reduce the skin's ability to produce vitamin D up to 98 percent. Vitamin D deficiency and insufficiency are linked to numerous health issues and affects 40- to 75 percent of people in the United States. Due to sunscreen use and indoor lifestyles, I am no longer surprised when I see even my patients from sunny Southern California with very low levels of vitamin D. Surprisingly, although sunscreen is supposed to protect us against skin cancer, a 2007 meta-analysis found that the use of sunscreen in areas above the sun-belt (above 40 degrees latitude) might actually contribute to the risk of melanoma—the most serious kind of skin cancer. A new sunscreen available in Australia called Solar-D allows vitamin D to be formed while providing protective SPF (sun protection factor), but its main active ingredients include several of the hormone-disrupting chemicals I just warned you about. If you are prone to burning, please continue to protect your skin, but I would also advise checking your vitamin D level to make sure you are not missing out on this important nutrient.

What about natural sunscreens? Numerous at-home recipes abound on the internet for natural oil-based sunscreens. While many oils such as olive or coconut oil do have some levels of SPF, most give a level of up to eight. This means that you can stay in the sun eight times longer than you normally would if you were not wearing any kind of SPF. The important thing here is to remember to re-apply. I do like the added benefit that some of these oils provide to your skin.

Other alternatives include using large-brimmed hats and UPF-rated clothes and swimsuits to cover yourself up and to minimize sun exposure when UV action is at its highest—between 10 a.m. and 2 p.m.

How to be Sun Savvy:

- **Check the EWG Guide to Sunscreens to see how your sunscreen scores and avoid potentially harmful ingredients such as: oxybenzone, avobenzone, nanoparticles, octinoxate, homosalate, octocrylene, retinyl palmitate, retinol, retinyl acetate, retinyl linoleate, retinoic acid, methylisothiozolinone (MI), and perfume/parfum/fragrance.**
- **Make sure your vitamin D level is sufficient by checking your blood 25-hydroxy vitamin D level and supplement with vitamin D3 (cholecalciferol) if needed.**
- **Avoid excessive sun exposure when UV levels are high (between 10 a.m. and 2 p.m.).**
- **Consider physical barriers to protect your skin if you are prone to burning including mineral sunscreens, wide-brimmed hats, and UPF-rated clothing.**

21. Wash Your Hands, but Forget the Antibacterial Soap

Hand washing with basic soap and water prevents the spread of infection and also prevents the transfer of toxic chemicals from your hands to your mouth, which can be especially important for children. While antibacterial soaps do kill bacteria and microbes, CDC and FDA advisory committees found no benefits over plain soap and water. So unless you are in a hospital or surgical center, there is really no advantage in using antibacterial products, and they actually may be causing harm.

After decades of use, an FDA ruling went into effect in 2017 banning nineteen ingredients found in thousands of over-the-counter antiseptic soaps and cosmetics. The chemicals, including triclosan and triclocarban, were found to pose possible health risks, cause environmental harm, and potentially worsen antibacterial resistance. The ban affects only FDA-regulated products such as soaps and cosmetics, so the chemicals can still be used, unlabeled, in building materials, clothing, toys, and other products. In addition, the FDA allowed Colgate-Palmolive to continue using triclosan in its Colgate Total toothpaste because studies found that it was more effective than fluoride alone.

Triclosan has been found to have endocrine-disrupting effects, to potentially increase liver toxicity, and to possibly contribute to bacterial resistance to antibiotics. Researchers at Johns Hopkins have also linked triclosan to increased risk of allergies and immune system disruption in children. Triclosan is absorbed into the body, can cross the placental barrier, and has been found widely in human urine and breast milk samples. It is not removed by wastewater treatment, so ends up in our water sources and is very toxic to aquatic life. In addition, when wastewater is treated with chlorine, the reaction with triclosan can form chlorinated by-products such as chloroform, which is categorized as a possible human carcinogen. Other antibacterial ingredients include triclocarban (noted to have similar effects as triclosan), benzethonium chloride (which can cause skin irritation and allergic reactions and can be highly toxic if ingested), or chloroxylenol (which can cause skin irritation or allergic reaction).

What About Hand Sanitizers?

If you like the convenience of waterless hand sanitizers, alcohol-based sanitizers are a better bet because they don't contain triclosan or triclocarban. But these products are not designed to remove dust and dirt, which is often how chemicals are transferred (particularly in children). And since the product is not washed off, all ingredients are left to fully absorb into your skin.

So if just washing with plain soap and water is good enough, why are these antibacterial products so popular? In the late 1800s, Louis Pasteur advanced the germ theory of disease and Joseph Lister promoted sanitation particularly in medical settings, opening our awareness to the fact that certain microbes can cause illness. Sanitation has been a cornerstone of preventing illness, but a broad-swath approach to killing organisms has taken it too far. More recently, scientists have learned what a valuable player our own microbiome is for our health, and attention has now turned to cultivating beneficial organisms with which we co-exist. The "Hygiene Hypothesis" suggests that a lack of early childhood exposure to infectious agents, symbiotic microorganisms, and parasites increases susceptibility to allergies by suppressing the immune system's natural development—dirt may actually be good for us!

Apart from soap, antimicrobial chemicals are put in wipes, dental products, cosmetics, shave gels and creams, hand gels, cutting boards, mattress pads, and a variety of home items. Before purchasing these items, I would seriously consider if the antibacterial action is truly necessary and what further effect it may have. Studies have confirmed that essential oils and herbal extracts are effective antimicrobial agents with less tendency to create organisms that are resistant to treatment.

Clean Your Hands Without Adding Toxins:
- **Wash your hands with soap and water.**
- **Avoid antimicrobial chemicals, particularly triclosan and triclocarban.**

22. Buy Your Kids Tight Pajamas

In the 1970s, 40 percent of Americans smoked, and cigarettes were a major cause of fires. So in 1975, California passed a law requiring the use of flame retardants in furniture (see Action Step 33), bedding, and even kids' pajamas. Since that time, flame-retardant chemicals have been widely used and are found to be fully penetrant and persistent in the environment. They off-gas into the air and bind to dust, and these compounds are hormonal disruptors, especially for the thyroid, and include carcinogens, skin irritants, and neurodevelopmental toxins. But since the 1970s the smoking rate has declined to less than 20 percent, and from 1980 to 2011 there was a 73 percent reduction in smoking-related fires, so are flame-retardant pajamas really necessary?

Chemicals used to make children's pajamas flame retardant include halogenated hydrocarbons (chlorine and bromine), inorganic flame retardants (antimony oxides), and phosphate-based compounds. Synthetic fabrics are either considered to be "inherently" flame resistant or are treated with flame retardants that can be chemically inserted into the polyester compound or treated after the material is woven. However, "inherently" flame resistant polyester textiles are manufactured with built-in fire retardants. Materials requiring chemical treatment include nylon, acetate, and triacetate. Materials not requiring treatment include most polyesters, modacrylic (Verel, SEF, Kanecaron); matrix (Cordelan); and vinyon (Leavil).

These fire-retardant chemicals are toxic, but the fear of catching fire might scare you into using them. What many do not realize is that a product treated with flame-retardant chemicals still can catch fire, and when it does, it gives off higher levels of toxic carbon monoxide, soot and smoke than an untreated product, and produces toxic dioxins and furans. Ironically, these toxic fumes are more likely to kill you than a burn, which means flame-retardant chemicals may actually make fires deadlier! There is pretty much no evidence showing that these chemicals make an impact in saving lives in a fire situation. In fact, many firefighter organizations are calling for a ban to using these types of flame retardants.

So why on earth would we want these toxic chemicals swaddling our children for nearly half the day? I remember becoming frustrated when I learned that the cute pajamas that my daughter picked out were tainted with toxic chemicals—most of the ones with popular cartoon characters are. Luckily, you can tell that they are because flame resistant garments are usually labeled "Flame Resistant."

Be Snug as a Bug

In 1997, snug-fitting, untreated cotton sleepwear became a legal alternative for children over nine months old (since most burn injuries result from children playing with fire and infants are less mobile, their sleepwear is exempt from the flame-resistant rule). All children's sleepwear above size nine months and up to size fourteen are required to be either "flame-resistant" or "tight-fitting." You may also note that there are some pajama-looking clothes that are labeled "Not Intended for Sleepwear," which means they are neither flame resistant nor tight fitting so they don't meet the requirements for official sleepwear—but who's to stop a kid from sleeping in a T-shirt and shorts? According to the Consumer Product Safety Commission (CPSC), loose-fitting sleepwear made of cotton or cotton blends are associated with 200 burn injuries every year, so just be aware that there can be a risk.

Tips to Find Less Toxic Children's Sleepwear:
- **Avoid clothing labeled "flame resistant" or that has been treated with Proban or Securest.**
- **Choose 100 percent organic cotton sleepwear that is tight fitting to minimize any potential risk.**

23. What Are You Wearing?

We already discussed flame-resistant clothing, but what does it mean if your clothes are stain-resistant, wrinkle-resistant, water-repellant, or "easy care?" While these treatments sound like a wish-come-true for those who don't iron or are prone to spilling, the chemicals (such as Teflon, other PFCs, and formaldehyde) and dyes in our clothing are another route for toxic exposure, causing skin reactions and shedding toxic dust.

Why Buy Organic Cotton and Wool Clothing?

There are a lot of wonderful natural fibers from which clothing can be made. Hemp is naturally insect resistant and therefore does not require treatment with pesticides. Flax and silk are also excellent fibers. But wool is often treated with pesticides to kill parasites. Cotton is the biggest textile in use, but much of it now is GMO cotton that is then treated heavily with herbicides. So if you are able to choose organic textiles, you will be exposed to fewer chemicals and also will be helping the environment.

Reduce Clothing Waste

In the United States, clothing has become so cheap that we have become used to just throwing it away. The EPA estimates that almost 13.1 million tons of textiles are thrown away every year, and while nearly half could be reused or recycled, only 15 percent actually are. This means that the average American throws away sixty-five to eighty pounds of textiles every year. So why is this so bad? For the most part, these textiles aren't biodegradable, so they end up sitting in landfills. In addition, the manufacturing of textiles uses a lot of water. For example, it takes about 700 gallons of water to make a cotton shirt, and 2,600 gallons to make a pair of jeans—most of it to grow the cotton. In addition, textiles are the fifth-largest contributor to carbon dioxide emission in the United States, a primary greenhouse gas contributing to climate change.

The creation of apparel is chemically intensive. In addition to special fabric treatments, from emissions to dyes, up to 2,000 chemicals are used in textile processing. Some in the apparel industry have decided to make a difference in the way they are impacting people and the environment, choosing to be more sustainable and environmentally responsible. Consumer products carrying the Bluesign label meet strict safety and environmental requirements based on five principles: resource productivity, consumer safety, water emission, air emission, and occupational health and safety. Bluesign helps to manage the chemical inputs to create a holistic system preventing contamination.

I'm not saying to never buy new clothes again, but bring awareness to your purchasing habits. I used to buy bags of clothes because they looked "okay" and the price was right, but I ended up having a closet full of clothes that I barely wore. Once I received some sage advice, I reduced my waste by deciding to only buy clothes that I loved and made me feel amazing or that I absolutely needed. And when you do purchase new clothes, choose wisely.

Tips to "Green" Your Wardrobe:
- **Choose natural fibers and organic cotton and organic wool if you can.**
- **Reduce clothing waste: buy less, re-use clothing by sharing or purchasing/selling at a re-seller, and recycle textiles if possible.**
- **Avoid fabrics which have been treated with stain or water repellant or that are wrinkle-resistant.**
- **Prewash all new clothes in Borax or a nontoxic detergent.**
- **Use a green dry-cleaner or air your dry-cleaned clothes out for forty-eight hours before bringing them into your home.**

24. If You Don't Smoke, Don't Start. If You Do Smoke, Attempt to Quit
Cigarette smoking exposes you and the people around you to hundreds of chemical compounds including combustion by-products, cancer-causing chemicals, and heavy metals. Indoor smoking is also the greatest source of solvent exposure. Since the Surgeon General's warning on the health dangers of cigarette smoking, smoking rates in the United States have declined significantly. However, people still smoke, and it is one of the most difficult habits to quit.

The good news is that there are many aids to help quit smoking, and research has shown that successful past quit attempts indicate future success at quitting. So even if you have quit before but started back up again, try, try, again.

Tips That Have Helped Many to Quit Smoking:

- Enlist the help of others. Tell your family, friends, co-workers, and health care providers and have them encourage you and keep you accountable.
- Surround yourself with non-smokers. It is easier to avoid smoking if you are not constantly tempted.
- Have alternatives at your fingertips. Do you need something for your mouth to do? Keep gum, tooth-picks, or water handy. Do you smoke when stressed or anxious? Learn alternative stress management techniques such as meditation and deep breathing. Try breath work and aromatherapy.
- Ask your health care provider about prescription and over-the-counter aids to help you quit.
- Consider acupuncture, which has been shown to help for many addictive habits.
- Cut down your amount if you are not yet ready to quit altogether.
- Establish a quit date and remove all smoking products and triggers, and thoroughly clean any areas where you usually smoke.

25. Align Yourself with the Rhythms of Nature

A daily routine that goes with the flow of nature can nurture your health, enhance detoxification, and bring balance into your life. Here are some basic principles that are used in Ayurveda:

Morning Routine

- Arise before or with the sun. Sleeping in can cause you to feel even more groggy.
- Eliminate wastes that have built up. Drink a glass of warm water. Urinate and move your bowels. Use a Neti Pot to cleanse your sinuses, particularly if you are prone to allergies or sinus trouble. Scrape your tongue and brush your teeth. I recommend using a metal tongue scraper

to gently scrape away any stuff that has accumulated on your tongue. Scrape from back to front about seven to fourteen times and then clean the tongue scraper. Brushing your tongue with a toothbrush just moves the coating around and does not remove it.

- Practice meditation and gentle stretching. Stretching before meditation can allow you to sit for a longer period of time. More vigorous physical activity can be performed any time after meditation.
- Bathe and perform an oil massage.
- Break your overnight fast mindfully (see Action Step 16 on Mindful Eating).

Daytime Routine

- Find time to get outside and be exposed to sunlight for at least fifteen minutes during the day to help keep your body-clock regulated.
- Move your body in an enjoyable way to get physical activity.
- Eat lunch mindfully. If you are able to take the time, make this the largest meal of the day, as your digestive capacity will be at its best.

Evening Routine

- Eat a lighter dinner. Digestion is strongest mid-day, and so your largest meal should be at that time. In the evening, our digestive power lessens, so it is best to eat lighter, easy to digest foods at this time.
- Go down with the sun. Follow the pattern of nature and begin to wind down. Dim your lights and minimize your screen time. Many studies have shown that the blue light emitted from electronic screens and lights can disrupt sleep. There are now apps, device settings, and special glasses that can help with the blue light balance

to minimize this effect. Instead of screen time, connect with loved ones or read uplifting books.

- Aim to be in bed with the lights out around 10 p.m. Not only will you get a good night's rest, but you will save electricity as well.

Ayurvedic Self-Massage

The ancient Ayurvedic technique of self-massage nourishes the body from head to toe, stimulates circulation and lymphatic drainage, softens the skin, and calms the mind. Warm some food-grade oil such as sesame or almond oil in a mug or with your hands and apply a small amount to the crown of your head, gently massaging the scalp. Then using small circular motions, apply oil to the rest of the body. Begin by massaging the face: the forehead, temples, cheeks, around the mouth and nose, jaw, and ears. Massage the neck and shoulders with circular motions. Then use long strokes to go along the long bones of the arms and circles around the elbow and wrist joints. Massage both hands including fingers and palms. Using broad strokes, massage the chest and the abdomen, moving up along the right side of the abdomen, then across, and down along the left side of the abdomen, following the path of the large intestine. Massage your back in broad strokes as well as you can. Using a circular motion, massage both hips. Then take long strokes to go along the long bones of the legs, with circles around the knees and ankles. Massage both feet all the way to the toes.

Optimize Your Ayurvedic Daily Routine
- Rise with the Sun
- Eliminate and cleanse (See Action Step 9)
- Stretch/Yoga
- Meditation

- Bathe
- Oil massage
- Breakfast
- Get outside
- Move
- Lunch largest
- Dinner lighter
- 10 p.m. in bed with lights out

26. Breathe

Most of us pay little attention to our breathing and may habitually have shallow breathing, which can add to chronic stress, tension, and even decreased cognitive function and brain fog. With our breath, we exhale carbon dioxide, removing acidity from the blood. Breathing also affects our parasympathetic nervous system (the rest and digest part of our nervous system), regulates heart rate variability (which is a measure of stress), influences the microbiome, and changes inflammatory markers. Just slowing our breath down and breathing more deeply can be helpful, and simple breathing techniques can help us optimize these effects.

Breathing Technique #1: Alternate Nostril Breathing

This technique quiets the mind and creates balance. Hold your right hand up, resting your pointer and middle fingers in between your eyebrows and place your thumb against your right nostril. Close your right nostril with your thumb, inhale through the left nostril. Close the left nostril with your ring finger, retain your breath for a brief moment. Release the thumb only, exhaling slowly through the right nostril. After exhaling completely, inhale through the right nostril keeping the ring finger on the left nostril. Close the right nostril with your thumb, pausing briefly and then release the ring finger, exhaling through the left nostril. You have now completed one cycle. Repeat for five to ten cycles.

Breathing Technique #2: Ujjayi Breath AKA Victorious Breath.

This technique is energizing and relaxing, assists with detoxification, and relieves agitation. With your mouth closed, slowly breathe in and out through your nose. As you exhale, gently constrict the muscles in the back of your throat so that you are making a noise that sounds like waves on the ocean. Continue to gently constrict the back of your throat as you inhale and exhale. If you have difficulty finding the sound of the breath, first try breathing with your mouth open, making a soft "ha" sound on the exhale as if you were trying to fog up a window. Once you have practiced a few times, try again with your mouth closed. Continue breathing in and out completely and deeply. Do this for three breaths up to several minutes.

Tips:
- **Make sure to use your lungs fully and deeply.**
- **Practice breathing techniques such as Alternate Nostril Breathing or Ujjayi Breath.**

27. Sweat

Sweating is one of our main detoxification routes, and often people with environmental toxicity are those who do not sweat easily, resulting in further toxic buildup. Studies have shown that therapeutic use of saunas can aid in detoxification of PCBs, pesticides, dioxins, and heavy metals. The act of sweating may be one of the many reasons why exercise and induced sweating traditions like saunas and sweat lodges are beneficial to our health. As for antiperspirants, I would advise against using them, as this prevents you from this natural way of detoxing. If you use deodorants, make sure they do not contain parabens or aluminum as those may be absorbed through the skin. An added bonus of fully cleansing your body and getting back into balance is a reduction in body odor, so if you detoxify and continue with a healthy lifestyle you may find you no longer need deodorant.

How to Detoxify Using a Sauna:

- **Check with your doctor**, especially if you are pregnant, have metal parts in your body, or take medications.
- **Mobilize chemicals first** by exercising and using a loofah or body brush to stimulate skin circulation. Sip a hot drink.
- **Start slow** in five- to ten-minute increments. **Build up your tolerance gradually** up to one or two thirty- to forty-minute sessions a day. **The goal is to induce profuse sweating.**
- **Either Far Infrared or traditional saunas can be used to induce sweating.** Far Infrared saunas allow for a lower overall temperature to be used (110 to 140° F versus 150 to 185° F for a traditional sauna) and may be more tolerable. Be cautious with saunas made from cedar wood as some people may be sensitive. Units that are made out of poplar or basswood hardwood are preferred. Be wary of the types of glues and adhesives that may be used in saunas as those can off-gas VOCs. Make sure you are not exposed to harmful EMFs.
- **Replenish water and electrolytes** (magnesium, zinc, calcium, potassium, and sodium) that are lost through sweat.
- **If blood pressure, pulse, or respiratory rate increase by ten points or more, get out of the sauna for the day. Stop immediately if you develop headache, nausea, fast heart rate, weakness, irregular heart rate, shortness of breath, dizziness, disorientation, muscle cramps, muscle spasms or twitching, or any adverse symptom. If you feel overheated, get out of the sauna and cool off in the shower.**

- **Keep drying off the sweat** with a towel and **shower** after you are finished to prevent reabsorption of toxins

28. Move Your Body

We all know that exercise is important for our health—burning calories, releasing endorphins, improving metabolism, and increasing our strength and endurance—but it is also important for detoxifying our body. Physical activity increases circulation of both blood and lymph and stimulates you to breathe more heavily and deeply. It makes you sweat and encourages bowels to eliminate. Physical exercise can also relax the mind and put you in the present moment. If you don't like going to the gym, find ways to increase your physical activity by incorporating more movement into your day. Park farther away and walk, take the stairs, stand rather than sit, walk for short five to ten minute stretches, perform physical chores (sweep instead of using a leaf blower, use a hand mower instead of a riding mower), and do things that you love where you are moving your body (play with your dog, go dancing, chase your toddler).

Balanced physical activity includes three components: aerobic or cardio exercises that increase heart rate and breathing (such as walking, swimming, or running); strength training (such as weights or resistance training) to build muscles; and stretching (such as static stretches, yoga, and Tai Chi), which increases flexibility and range of motion. Depending on your body constitution and needs, different types of physical activity may be more or less beneficial, but it is important for everyone to incorporate all three components.

We can further support our detoxification processes by stimulating lymphatic movement. Lymph is the fluid in our body that carries waste, debris, toxins, and unhealthy cells to be processed. Performing twists and bends in hatha yoga massages the internal organs and facilitates flow. Massage can also stimulate lymph circulation (see Action Step 25 for instructions on performing an Ayurvedic self-massage). Rebounding, jumping, and doing hot-cold plunges also boost blood and lymph circulation.

How to Do a Hot-Cold Plunge

Our skin contains miles of blood vessels that relax and dilate with heat and contract with cold. When relaxation and contraction are alternated, your skin pumps more blood, increasing circulation to that area. In the shower, turn water on as hot as you can tolerate for one minute and then as cold as you can take for one minute. Repeat four to five times. Make sure to end on cold.

Yoga for Digestion, Elimination, and Detoxification

Yoga postures can improve muscle tone, flexibility, strength, and stamina. The sun salutation sequence allows you to use all of the major muscle groups and move all of your major joints. Certain postures can also facilitate detoxification, including stretching, folds, and gentle twists. My favorites include child's pose, lunges, eagle, plank, bow, seated forward fold, reclining knee-to-chest, plow, and gentle twists such as seated twist, revolved chair pose, lunging prayer twist, twisting triangle, and twisting half-moon.

Chapter 7:
Living in It: Home,
Garage, and Yard

"If it looks clean and smells clean, it may be toxic."
— *Walter Crinnion, N.D.*

You don't have to live near a smokestack or gas leak to have toxins lurking in your home. Chances are, many of the products you use in everyday life have substances that can potentially cause harm. From cleaning supplies to furnishings to pesticides and building materials, we are inundated with a stunning array of chemicals in our homes.

Detoxifying this area of your life can take significant time, effort, and may require spending some money. Replacing certain items may be necessary for some people, particularly if the item is particularly noxious or a person is especially sensitive or already ill. However, many of the following tips can actually save money by simplifying and using inexpensive, natural cleaning products.

In this section you will learn how to detoxify your cleaning products, how to minimize toxic exposures from dust and air, and what to look for in your children's toys. You will learn what home furnishings might be shedding toxic dust, how your shower may be exposing you to carcinogens, and how to choose the least toxic flooring and paints for your home. We will also explore the topic of toxic mold, which can be an invisible but serious threat. Then we take it outside to minimize exposures in your garage and yard. I've also included some tips on backyard composting to improve the quality of your soil and reduce food waste.

When you become aware of these areas to improve upon, you can incorporate changes when you are able to (or when you need to). Because your toxic load is an accumulation of all of the exposures in your life, each small step can make a difference.

29. What's That Smell?

What makes products from cleaning supplies to perfumes have a scent? Unless your product is 100 percent organic, chances are it is a combination of chemicals labeled as "fragrance." In 2009, about one-third of Americans had experienced sensitivity to scented products and 19 percent reported headaches or breathing difficulties when exposed to air fresheners or deodorizers. Although many people are sensitive to "fragrance," manufacturers insist on keeping their formulations as trade secrets and rarely disclose the identity of the chemicals used to create their fragrances. And it is the manufacturers themselves within the International Fragrance Association that self-regulate the safety of their products. Other products, such as laundry detergents and air fresheners, fall under the Consumer Products Safety Commission, which currently does not actively screen fragrances for safety nor require labeling.

Independent analysis of products with "fragrance" has revealed undisclosed chemicals including endocrine disruptors, allergens, and other hazardous chemicals. Some of these include ones which have been flagged with a "warning" or "danger" label by the UN, categorized as possible human carcinogens by the IARC, or banned from cosmetics in the EU. Many air fresheners are full of solvents which are neurotoxic. In fact, some even have a drug-abuse warning on the can because they are so high in solvents they may be abused.

Tips for Getting a Clean Scent Without Getting Toxic:

- **Use essential oils as fragrance. Diffusers can be used to spread the aroma in your environment or you can burn a nontoxic candle made from soy or beeswax with essential oils for aroma. Be careful when using essential oils topically, as some people may be sensitive.**
- **Some companies make nontoxic deodorizers such as Ava Anderson Non-Toxic Pet Deodorizer.**
- **Moso bags use charcoal to absorb unpleasant odors.**
- **Use an air filter (see Action Step 31).**
- **Use baking soda and vinegar, which are safe deodorizers.**

The Magic of Baking Soda and Vinegar

- Sprinkle baking soda over rugs, carpets, upholstery, mattresses, and pet beds. Allow it to sit for fifteen minutes, then vacuum thoroughly.
- Deodorize garbage pails and compost bins by washing with white vinegar and then sprinkling baking soda on the bottom of the pail.
- Deodorize sneakers and gym bags by filling an old pair of socks with two tablespoons of baking soda. Tie the top of each sock into a knot and place them inside your sneakers or gym bag. Replace the baking soda monthly.
- Freshen laundry: Sprinkle ½ cup baking soda into the washing machine to neutralize the smell of musty towels. If wet laundry has been sitting in the machine

---

too long, rerun the wash with a cup of vinegar or baking soda.

- Deodorize your sink by pouring ½ cup of baking soda down the drain. Allow to sit for a few minutes, then rinse with warm water. For extra-strength odors, rinse with 2 cups of white vinegar instead of water.

30. "Green" Your Cleaning Supplies

Many of the products that we use for cleaning contain ingredients linked to asthma, cancer, reproductive toxicity, hormone disruption, neurotoxicity, and other adverse health effects. An EPA study revealed that toxic chemicals in household cleaners are three times more likely to cause cancer than outdoor air. Often it is difficult to find out what exactly is in those products, as the government doesn't require that cleaning products carry a list of ingredients or even require that products and ingredients are tested for health and safety. Most cleaning products rely on petroleum-based surfactants, solvents, and other chemicals. As the chemicals are washed down the drain, they also end up affecting fish and marine ecosystems.

There are many natural and economical products that do a great job at cleaning. Lemon, vinegar, salt, and baking soda are staples. Hydrogen peroxide, rubbing alcohol, and castile soap can also be helpful. As you run out of your current products, switch over to more nontoxic alternatives. Until then, store your chemical-laden products in airtight containers so that they don't pollute your indoor air.

General Advice:

- **Beware of "greenwashing."** Greenwashing is when products tout a natural, eco-friendly, or otherwise "green" claim but still contain harmful chemicals. Use EWG's Guide to Healthy Cleaning to see what's in your cleaners and to find safer alternatives. Certain certifications may indicate safer, eco-friendly products which have been independently tested, such as Green Seal and EcoLogo.

- **Check warning labels**. If a product has a warning label, consider if there might be a safer alternative. If you must use the product, protect yourself with gloves and other precautions, and ventilate by opening a window or running an exhaust fan.
- **Use nontoxic options like baking soda and vinegar and skip some of the biggest hazards** like air fresheners, oven cleaners, and drain cleaners. See Clean Kitchen Tips for less toxic alternatives.
- **Keep kids away** from toxic products, as they are more vulnerable to toxic chemicals. If they want to help, let them clean with soap and water, not toxic cleaners.
- **Less is more**. Dilute your cleaning supplies and use only what's needed to get the job done.
- **Avoid "antibacterial" products** (see Action Step 21).
- **Never mix bleach** with ammonia, vinegar, or other acids, as these combinations can produce deadly gases.
- **Be careful with pine and citrus oil cleaners** as some people may be sensitive, and avoid using these cleaners especially on smoggy days when ingredients can react with ozone to produce cancer-causing formaldehyde.
- **Dispose of your old toxic products safely** by contacting your local waste management company to find out how to throw away household hazardous waste. Do not pour cleaning supplies down the drain as some of the ingredients can harm wildlife as well as people.

Clean Kitchen Tips:
- **Removing stuck/burned food**: After removing the food, but while the pan is still hot, slowly pour in a 50:50 mixture of vinegar and water and allow it to bubble. You may need to turn on low heat if it doesn't bubble. Scrape the bottom of the pan with a wooden spoon or

a food-safe plastic scraper. If this doesn't do the trick, pour baking soda on whatever is still stuck and then pour vinegar over the area. Allow to bubble and then scrape off, then rinse and wash.

- **Degreaser:** Pour a small amount of vinegar or lemon juice on greasy pans or dishes to help dissolve buildup.
- **Oven cleaner**: Mix a solution of baking soda, water, and vinegar in an ovenproof bowl. Apply the mixture with a sponge to the soiled areas of the oven and place the bowl with the remainder of the mixture onto the oven rack (I have found that this part can be optional but helps when the oven is really a mess). Turn the oven to 200° F for forty-five minutes. Wipe the soiled areas with a damp sponge. Avoid using the self-cleaning feature on ovens, as this can heat the materials to extremely high temperatures releasing toxic fumes (see Action Step 13).
- **Unclog a drain:** First remove as much liquid and solid as possible. Pour ½ to 1 cup baking soda directly into the drain followed by ½ to 1 cup vinegar poured in slowly. Wait fifteen to thirty minutes. Then run hot water for one minute followed by cold water for one minute. You may need to repeat and consider doing regularly for drains that clog often.
- **Clean counters** frequently and change out **sponges** frequently. Sponges can be cleaned by soaking in full-strength vinegar for five minutes, then rinse well or boil in water for five minutes.
- **Countertop disinfectant**: Mix a 50:50 rubbing alcohol and water solution in a spray bottle and use it to wipe down countertops. Add a few drops of essential oil if you want a scent.
- Take out the garbage regularly to avoid germs, pests, and bad odors.

- **Odor eliminator**: Sprinkle baking soda or a mixture of baking soda and water and allow to sit for at least one to two hours. This can be used in food containers, trash cans, and even on upholstery (test a small area first)—just vacuum it up after an hour.

Clean Bathroom Tips:
- **All-purpose cleaner**: Mix together ¼ cup baking soda, ½ cup white vinegar, and the juice of one lemon. Rinse well with warm water after use.
- **Toilets**: Scrub with baking soda and water instead of an acidic toilet-bowl cleaner. Or pour 1 cup of full-strength white vinegar into the toilet and scrub well with a toilet brush. Wait one hour and then flush.
- **Showers:** Wipe down showers after each use to prevent mold and mildew. Clean **grout and tile** with a paste of ½ cup baking soda and 2 tablespoons dish soap or liquid castile soap. For mild bleaching and disinfecting, add 1 tablespoon hydrogen peroxide.
- **Dissolve soap scum**: Mix ½ cup salt in 1 cup warm water. Add 2 cups vinegar and place mixture in a spray bottle. Use the mixture and scrub with a sponge, then rinse.
- **Clean the air**: Instead of toxic air fresheners, open a window, run a fan, set out a box of baking soda or a Moso bag, or use all natural botanical sprays, scented nontoxic candles, or essential oil diffusers. (See Action Step 31 for more details on cleaner air, which also details houseplants that help clean the air.)
- **Unclog a drain**: See Kitchen Tips on how to unclog a drain. A mechanical snake can also be helpful to dislodge hair.
- **Windows and mirror cleaner**: Mix one part vinegar and one to two parts water. Spray or apply with a sponge and wipe with old newspaper or microfiber cloth.

Clean Floor and Furniture Tips:

- **Sweep and vacuum** frequently to remove dust (see Action Step 32). Consider getting a HEPA vacuum, particularly if allergies are an issue.
- **Mop** with a dilute vinegar solution (e.g., ¼ cup vinegar in 1 quart of water).
- **Dust** with a soft cloth and skip dusting sprays.
- **Furniture polish**: Mix together 2 tablespoons vinegar or lemon juice with 6 tablespoons olive or canola oil. Shake well. Dampen a clean, soft cloth with the mixture. Test on a small area first.

Laundry Tips:

- **Choose unscented laundry detergent and fabric softener.** You can add ¼ cup of vinegar or baking soda to the rinse cycle as a fabric softener or use felted wool dryer balls. Products with vegetable-based surfactants and softeners may also be better. Skip toxic dryer sheets.
- **Try plant-based detergents** to avoid conventional detergents made with petroleum products, fragrances, and phosphates, which are harmful for local waterways.
- **Stain remover**: For stains, use borax, washing soda, lemon juice, hydrogen peroxide, white vinegar, or non-chlorine bleach.
- **Hang laundry** to dry if you are able.

31. Care for Your Air

While most people are familiar with outdoor air pollution—such as smog from industry and vehicle exhaust, which are important to address for health and climate change—studies indicate that the majority of air pollutants in your lungs actually come from indoor rather than outdoor air. We are exposed to volatile organic compounds (VOCs) that are released from our furnishings, home construction materials, and products that we use in daily life. We are also exposed to dust in our carpets, on our furniture, and in the air, which becomes contaminated with a variety of toxic materials. To make things worse, many homes today are airtight to conserve energy, and without cross-ventilation, levels of indoor air pollutants tend to stay higher. The most common indoor air pollutants today come from mothballs, deodorizers, plastic, foam rubber, insulation, tobacco smoke, off-gassing from dry-cleaning, paint, cleaning products, steam from chlorinated water, and molds.

Tackling Sources of Indoor Air Pollution:

- Replace products containing synthetic fragrance such as deodorizers, air fresheners, laundry detergents, and dryer sheets with nontoxic options (see Action Step 29).
- Green your cleaning supplies (see Action Step 30).
- Choose less toxic products when purchasing furniture (see Action Steps 33 and 35).
- Replace your vinyl shower curtain with a fabric one (see PVCs in Action Step 39).
- Choose no-VOC paint and no-VOC glue for carpets and flooring (see Action Step 39).
- Air out your dry cleaning before bringing it in the house to avoid being exposed to chemicals such as perchloroethylene (PERC). Solvents used for dry-cleaning may continue to off-gas from your clothing for over two weeks after you have removed the plastic wrap. Remove the plastic bag and hang any dry-cleaned clothes outside (or in a mudroom or garage) to air out for at least forty-eight hours before wearing or hanging in your closet. Less toxic "green" or organic dry-cleaner options exist that use liquid carbon dioxide (CO_2), silicon-based solvent, or "wet cleaning"" which uses water and nontoxic detergents in high-tech machines.

- Don't wear shoes indoors as this will track outside contaminants inside the home.
- Dust and clean your home regularly. Wash sheets and blankets weekly in hot water.
- Don't allow smoking indoors. If you smoke, wash your hands and change your clothes as soon as possible when coming indoors (see Action Step 24).
- Avoid living near a freeway if possible. Close windows during peak traffic hours.
- Natural gas may be a problem for some people. Ventilate when cooking and check fireplace, stove, furnace, and garage for leaks.
- Clean up mold and fix water leaks promptly and properly (see Action Step 40).

Cleaning the Air

- Open windows and run exhaust fans regularly to ventilate. Even ventilating for thirty minutes a day can make a difference.
- Change air filters on your forced air system every one to three months (look for MERV rating of 12 or higher) and clean the vents. An air filter with a MERV of 7 will help with dust and higher ratings will help with off-gassing, smaller sized particles, tobacco smoke, and microbes.
- For room air purifiers, choose one that uses a fan to push or pull the air through a HEPA filter and that will clean the air in a specified space (the width x length x height of your room). A high quality air purifier filters the air in the space about every twenty minutes. The bedroom is a good place to start as most people spend a large amount of time there. Avoid air purifiers that use ozone, which is itself an air pollutant and can affect the lungs. See Resources for recommendations.

Let Plants Clean Your Air

A NASA study found that certain houseplants can filter out common VOCs and improve indoor air quality. If you are mold sensitive, I would advise against this, as there is a potential for mold growth in the soil.

Helpful Houseplants

Aloe *Aloe vera*	This easy-to-grow, sun-loving succulent helps clear formaldehyde and benzene from a variety of household sources. Beyond its air-clearing abilities, the gel inside the leaves is also helpful for minor cuts and burns.
Spider plant *Chlorophytum comosum*	A resilient plant with rich foliage and tiny white flowers that is pet-safe. This helps remove benzene, formaldehyde, carbon monoxide, and xylene. It thrives in cool-to-average home temperatures, dry soil, and bright indirect sunlight.
Gerbera daisy *Gerbera jamesonii*	Removes trichloroethylene (which may be released from dry-cleaned clothes) and benzene. It does well with at least six hours of direct sunlight daily. Mist leaves a couple of times a week, and make sure the soil is well-drained.
Snake plant *Sansevieria trifasciata 'Laurentii'*	With sharp leaves, this plant is also known as mother-in-law's tongue and is one of the best for handling formaldehyde. It can thrive in low light and humid conditions, so it is ideal for the bathroom.

Golden pothos aka Devil's Ivy *Scindapsus aures*	Fast-growing vine that does well as a hanging basket and helps with form-aldehyde. It needs bright, indirect light. This is a poisonous plant and should be kept away from small chil-dren and pets
Chrysanthemum *Chrysantheium morifolium*	Helps to filter out benzene. It does well in bright light and requires direct sunlight for buds to open. Choose a floral mum instead of garden variety, which is for outdoors.
Red-edged dracaena *Dracaena marginata*	Helps filter xylene, trichloroethylene, and formaldehyde. It grows slowly but can reach fifteen feet tall, so it may be best for a room with high ceilings and moderate sunlight. Purple-red edges on ribbon-like green leaves
Warneck dracaena *Dracaena deremensis 'Warneckii'*	Known for its white stripes along the edges of its leaves, this dracaena grows inside easily and can reach a height of twelve feet. It helps with benzene, formaldehyde, and trichloroethylene.
Weeping fig *Ficus benjamina*	This ficus removes formaldehyde, benzene, and trichloroethylene. It does best in bright, indirect light.
English ivy *Hedera helix*	This plant filters formaldehyde. It does best with moist soil and four or more hours of direct sunlight each day.
Chinese evergreen *Aglaonema Crispum 'Deborah'*	Easy to care for, this plant thrives in low light and humid air. It helps with a variety of air pollutants. If your air is too dry, mist the leaves occasionally.

Bamboo palm aka reed palm *Chamaedorea sefritzii*	One of the best plants for handling benzene and trichloroethylene. This small palm produces flowers and small berries and prefers humidity, bright, indirect light, and well-drained soil, growing to about five to seven feet tall.
Heart leaf philodendron *Philodendron oxycardium*	A climbing vine, this removes VOCs such as formaldehyde and is low-maintenance, requiring indirect light. Avoid with children and pets as it is toxic when eaten.
Peace lily *Spathiphyllum*	This easy-care plant is also beautiful and does well in shade with weekly watering. It filters formaldehyde, benzene, trichloroethylene, toluene, and xylene.

32. Banish Your Dust Bunnies

Not only is dust allergenic and unsightly, it also is a source of exposure to toxic chemicals. Indoor dust becomes attached to particles from disintegrated products in your home, from upholstered furniture and electronics with flame retardants, vinyl shower curtains and carpets with PVCs and solvents, phthalates from your kid's toys, formaldehyde from your furniture and clothing, lead from paint, as well as particles coming in on your shoes from the outdoors like pesticides and herbicides. A study by the Silent Spring Institute identified sixty-six endocrine-disrupting compounds as well as other chemicals in household dust. With all of these toxic chemicals accumulating in one place, it is a very good reason to banish your dust bunnies.

The potential effect on young children is even more concerning because they are more vulnerable to toxic exposures due to an immature detoxification system as well as the large impact that small amounts of toxins can exert at critical developmental periods. In addition, children ingest or inhale more dust than adults since they spend lots of time on or very near the floor and often put dusty hands and toys in their mouths.

Take measures to reduce the toxic dust load in your home by avoiding products that can shed toxic particles and by cleaning often. If you are dust sensitive, consider asking someone else to do the dusty cleaning. As an added bonus, these tips also improve the air quality in your home.

Floor Care:
- **Leave your shoes at the door** and use a natural doormat at each entrance. Shoes are a common way we bring outdoor pollutants inside. Clean your pet's paws when they come back into the house as well.
- **Vacuum frequently** and use a vacuum fitted with a HEPA filter to trap small particles and remove contaminants and allergens. This is important as these particles may actually be recirculated into the air if using a regular vacuum. Change the filter as recommended to keep it working well. Vacuum upholstered furniture as well.
- **Wet mop** uncarpeted floors frequently to prevent dust from accumulating.
- **Seal cracks and crevices** to prevent dust from accumulating in hard-to-reach places.
- **Pay special attention to areas where young children crawl, sit, and play.**
- **When you create dust, clean up quickly and thoroughly.**

Furniture and Electronics:
- **Buy furniture made from natural materials and avoid fire retardants and other chemical treatments.**
- **Replace upholstered furniture** made with foam between 1970 and 2005, as they likely contain PBDEs.

157

Do this especially if the covering is ripped or foam is misshapen or breaking down. If you can't replace these items, try to keep the covers intact and vacuum frequently to remove dust particles.

- **Wipe furniture and electronic equipment** with a damp cloth or microfiber cloth to grab onto dust. Skip synthetic sprays and wipes when you dust, which can contain additional chemicals.
- **Choose home electronics without PBDE flame retardants.** There are manufacturers who no longer use them in some products, so ask before you buy.

Trap the Dust with a Filter:
- **Consider a high efficiency "HEPA-filter" air cleaner for individual rooms. See Resources for Action Step 31.**
- **Use high-quality filters for your forced-air heating or cooling system** and change them frequently to keep them working well. Look for higher MERV ratings (at least 7).

33. Fire the Flame Retardants
In the 1970s, as manufacturers increasingly put fast-burning synthetic materials and plastics in their products and when 40 percent of Americans were smokers, the use of organohalogen flame retardants (OFRs) in products increased. Since that time, flame retardants have been commonly added to furniture containing polyurethane foam, including couches, upholstered chairs, futons, and carpet padding. A large couch can have up to two pounds in its foam cushions! They have also been added to mattresses and children's sleepwear (see Action Steps 22 and 34) as well as other children's products such as car seats. Some TVs, remotes, cell phones, and other electronics, as well as building materials, also contain chemical flame retardants. All of this amounts to approximately 1.5 million tons of flame retardants used globally every year.

But there are several problems with flame retardants. The first is that they do not necessarily improve fire safety. In fact, the CDC itself reported in their Fire Death and Injuries Fact Sheet that most victims of fires die from smoke or toxic gases and not from burns. And when flame retardants burn, they release toxic gases such as dioxins and furans and increase the amount of carbon monoxide and hydrogen cyanide released. The International Association of Firefighters reports a link to high levels of cancer among firefighters.

The second issue is that flame retardants are associated with serious health problems including cancer, reproductive problems, neurodevelopmental issues, hormone disruption, and lowered immunity. When they are sprayed into fabrics and foams used in furniture, bedding, and clothing, the chemicals end up being attached to dust particles that leach out and disperse into the air and may end up being ingested and inhaled, and children are particularly affected.

The bottom line is that these flame retardant chemicals end up in us, with levels of these chemicals in the blood of adults having doubled every two to five years between 1970 and 2004. More than 97 percent of US residents have OFRs in their blood. Babies in the United States are born with the highest recorded concentrations of flame retardants in the world. These chemicals have been measured in breast milk and so find their way into children's bodies in yet another way. Children are especially at-risk because they have immature detoxification systems and have greater exposure to household dust than adults, and children who play indoors most often have the highest blood levels of flame retardants (three to five times higher than their parents). Flame retardant chemicals are persistent and have become ubiquitous; they are detected in the blood of remote Arctic polar bears and in the bark of trees ranging from Tasmania to Indonesia. They also end up in food, particularly fatty items like butter, peanut butter, bacon, and salmon.

Amid growing concerns about the potential risks posed by flame retardants to human health and the environment, a revised flammability standard was put into effect in 2014 (TB117-2013), allowing for fire safety to be met without flame retardant chemicals and requiring furniture companies to label whether their product contains flame retardants or not. Naturally fire-resistant fabrics (like wool) have been shown to be much more effective at preventing fires in real world conditions. Under this standard, certain children's products were exempted from California's furniture flammability standard, however, car seats must still comply with the federal motor vehicle flammability standard and continue to contain flame retardants.

In response to a petition filed by leading consumer, healthcare, firefighter, and science groups, in September 2017 the US Consumer Product Safety Commission (CPSC) initiated steps to ban OFRs, calling on manufacturers to voluntarily eliminate these compounds from consumer products and urging both retailers and consumers to "obtain assurances" from companies that their products are OFR-free. Because it could take years for a ban to take effect, the commission also issued an emphatic warning to consumers, especially pregnant women and young children, to avoid products containing OFRs in the meantime.

Firing Your Flame Retardants:

- **Be aware of children's products that you purchase and choose products which are free of flame retardants if possible.** Choose products whose labels read "contains no added flame retardants."
- **Check furniture labels.** A California law requires all new upholstered furniture sold in the state to include a visible label that makes clear whether flame retardant chemicals were added. Consumers outside the state should also look for this label. If you can't find it, ask

a salesperson or contact the manufacturer directly for more information.

- **Avoid products made with polyurethane foam, which tends to contain high concentrations of OFRs.** Furniture that does not contain polyurethane foam or that was made or reupholstered prior to 1975 usually does not contain flame retardant chemicals. In addition to flame retardant treatment, polyurethane foam also off-gasses VOCs, such as solvents.
- **If you want to know if flame retardants are in a polyurethane foam product that you already own,** you can send a sample of it to Duke University, where researchers will analyze it for free. See Resources section for details.
- **Naturally flame-resistant textiles include 100 percent wool, 100 percent cotton or flannel, and leather.** Kevlar is a synthetic fire-resistant material that so far appears to be nontoxic.
- **Check if your electronics have flame retardants or not.**
- **Vacuum and wash hands frequently to reduce exposure to toxic dust.**
- **In addition, skip optional stain treatments on carpets and furniture to avoid PFCs.**

34. Are You Sleeping with the Enemy? Find Out What's in Your Mattress.

We spend about one-third of our lives in our beds (even more for kids), so it is important to understand exactly what we are sleeping with. Flame retardants? Volatile organic compounds from petroleum-based products? Mold? Several years ago when we were in the market for a new mattress, I was surprised to find out that mattress manufacturers are not required to label or disclose which chemicals their mattresses contain. When I called several of the major mattress companies and explained that I had chemical sensitivities and would like to know what their mattress was made of, all of them refused, saying it was proprietary information.

Foam mattresses seem to be a particular problem for some, as they are made from petroleum and can emit VOCs and lead to buildup of solvent levels in blood. This can create symptoms, particularly in those who are genetically susceptible to being unable to clear solvents or in those with a high toxic load in general. I have had many patients develop health problems after getting a new memory foam mattress. One hundred percent organic natural latex mattresses are an excellent alternative. But beware of latex mattresses that are blended with synthetic latex which is also derived from petroleum. A mattress labelled "natural latex" may contain only 50 percent natural latex and may be blended with polyurethane foam and treated with VOCs. So be sure to look for mattresses that specify that they are made from 100 percent natural latex. Biofoam is another marketing ploy that uses soy or plant foam but typically contains less than 20 percent plant material with the rest made of mostly polyurethane (a petroleum-based material that emits VOCs).

You will also want to look at what the mattress covering is made with to avoid flame retardants. In addition, vinyl and phthalates may be present in children's mattresses and should be avoided. In the 1970s, cigarettes were a main cause of mattress fires leading to a requirement that certain products be treated with flame retardants which are now known to be hazardous to human health (see Action Step 33). Although manufacturers have shifted away from use of toxic PBDE, most do not disclose exactly what it is they are currently using as a chemical flame retardant. A new law as of 2014 allows manufacturers to meet new flammability standards without use of toxic chemicals, so look for the TB117-2013 label on new mattresses to see if it contains fire retardants or not.

Mattresses covered in cotton and wool are an excellent option that is naturally flame resistant. Choose 100 percent organic cotton to avoid insecticides, fungicides, and chemical fertilizers used for conventionally grown cotton. Wool may also be a source of exposure to pesticides and chemicals and also should be 100 percent organic if possible.

If electromagnetic fields concern you, you may also consider avoiding metal springs in your mattress.

Tips for a Healthy Bed:

- **Avoid memory foam, biofoam, or any mattress that doesn't specifically identify what is in it.**
- **If choosing natural latex, make sure it is 100 percent natural latex.**
- **Choose naturally flame-resistant materials such as 100 percent organic cotton or wool mattress coverings.**
- **Avoid vinyl coverings on children's beds.**
- **Look for third party certifications such as GreenGuard, Oeko-Tex, Global Organic Textile Standard (GOTS), and organic agricultural standards. Don't trust certifications created by the industry or its trade associations such as National Association of Organic Mattress Industry or CertiPUR.**
- **While you're at it, choose pillows made out of natural materials such as feathers, wool, cotton, buckwheat, or 100 percent natural latex foam.**

35. Don't Finish Your Furniture

Glues, finishes, foam, fabric treatments, and flame retardants can all make your furniture a source of toxic gases and dusts. Old furniture may have off-gassed after a few years, but be sure to use a HEPA vacuum cleaner or steam cleaner to remove any current dust. When purchasing new furniture, consider going for greener options. Ikea is well known to have more eco-friendly options, but you still have to pay attention to the materials going into the specific product. More furniture companies are also offering less toxic furnishings, so here's what to avoid and what to look for.

Glues in particleboard, chipboard, pressed wood, and plywood to make wood and upholstered furniture can emit formaldehyde and VOCs for years. There are some formaldehyde-free furniture glues out there, so ask what type is used when purchasing new furniture. You will also want to pay attention to internal pieces (drawers, backs, and bottoms) as they may be made of particleboard or plywood. Wood furniture finishes, particularly those that are oil-based, may also emit chemicals. Opt for untreated, natural woods that are unfinished.

For upholstered furniture, avoid polyurethane foam, which may emit VOCs like solvents. In addition, foam and covering fabrics are often treated with flame retardants, stain repellant, and waterproofing, which can off-gas and create toxic dust (see Action Steps 32 and 33). Choose 100 percent natural latex or natural fibers (cotton, wool, hemp, etc.) for the fill and untreated, natural fibers for the covering.

Tips for Detoxing Your Furniture:
- **Choose formaldehyde-free, unfinished furniture made from natural fibers and materials.**
- **Refrain from added treatments such as stain-resistance, waterproofing, and flame retardants.**
- **If you have furniture that is potentially releasing toxic gases or dusts, make sure to dust frequently and use an air filter and/or plants that clean the air naturally.**

36. Filter Your Shower, if Not Your Whole House.
Many people focus on drinking purified water, but we can also be exposed through the water that we bathe with. As one who loves a nice hot shower, I was really surprised to learn that the worst chlorine exposure in daily life is via inhalation in the

shower. Chlorine has been used for decades to sanitize drinking water and as a home cleaner, but adverse health effects are well known. Chlorine is an irritant, harmful to eyes, skin, respiratory passages, and lungs. It also is a free-radical initiator that can contribute to arteriosclerosis as well as various types of cancers of the rectum and bladder. Chloramine is a combination of chlorine and ammonia that is also used as a disinfecting agent in water treatment and causes similar effects. When chlorine is used in water treatment, it combines with organic matter to form compounds called trihalomethanes (THMs)—also known as disinfectant by-products (DBPs)—which can be even more harmful than chlorine. Chloroform is one of the most common THMs formed and is a known carcinogen. The amount of THMs in drinking water are regulated, however, it is estimated that at least one thousand water districts in the United States have levels which exceed the regulated amount. These water disinfection by-products are associated with an increased risk of cancer and possible adverse effects during pregnancy.

Although our bodies can handle much of the chlorine from treated drinking water, taking a shower can increase risk of inhalation of THMs and other DBPs. It is said that the dose of chloroform from a ten-minute shower is equal to, if not greater than, a dose from ingesting two liters of water.

In addition to these health risks, chloramine increases leaching of lead from pipes. And to make matters worse, combining chloramines with fluoride (hydrofluorosilicic acid, or HFSA) that has been added to most water supplies makes a potent combination that extracts even more lead. In fact, fluorosilic acid has been used for industrial purposes as a solvent for lead and other heavy metals because of its particular affinity for lead. HFSA is a by-product of the phosphate fertilizer industry, a hazardous waste that is collected to avoid polluting the air and water and then sold to municipal water districts to use as fluoride treatment. HFSA often also contains arsenic. Wait, what? Who ever heard of disposing of a hazardous waste by administering it to our citizens as a treatment? Well, unfortunately, it is happening all the time.

Alarmingly, these lead-loving fluoridation additives are not the same form of fluoride that is found in toothpaste which is usually simple sodium fluoride salt. As shown in research, the main benefits of fluoride for preventing dental caries or cavities are derived from surface application on teeth, not from ingestion. In contrast, a substantial and growing body of peer-reviewed science suggests that ingesting fluoride in tap water does not provide any additional dental benefits over those offered by fluoride toothpaste and may in fact present serious health risks. Ingestion of fluoride causes dental and skeletal fluorosis and gastrointestinal irritation as well as acute toxicity with overdose. Based on epidemiologic studies, it was also classified as a neurotoxin in a 2014 *The Lancet* article by Dr. Philippe Grandjean and Dr. Philip Landrigan. Fluoride has also been linked to behavioral disorders, lower IQ, and alteration in metabolism of testosterone. These risks are especially significant for infants and young children, and parents are encouraged to use fluoride-free bottled water to reconstitute concentrated or powdered infant formula to avoid excess fluoride ingestion.

Chromium-6

In 2016, the EWG released a report that chromium-6, the cancer-causing chemical made famous by the Erin Brockovich story, is present at higher-than-recommended levels in the tap water supplying more than 200 million Americans in all 50 states. And that number may underestimate exposure, as this does not account for smaller utilities and private wells. Although the National Toxicology Program found almost ten years ago that chromium-6 caused cancer in rodents when ingested, there are still no federal regulations on chromium-6 in drinking water and no federal requirements for regular monitoring of chromium-6 in tap water. Chromium-6 can cause lung cancer, liver damage, reproductive problems, and developmental harm. Greater risk may occur in certain groups including infants, children, people who take antacids, and people with poor liver function.

There are two main types of chromium compounds. Chromium-3 (trivalent chromium) is a naturally occurring compound and an essential human nutrient. Chromium-6 (hexavalent chromium) also occurs naturally, but it is also manufactured for use in steel making, chrome plating, manufacturing dyes and pigments, preserving leather and wood, and lowering the temperature of water in cooling towers of electrical power plants. It is present in the ash from coal-burning power plants, which is typically dumped into unlined pits and can threaten water supplies and private wells. Some methods of treating water supplies to remove other contaminants may actually increase levels of chromium-6, making the problem worse.

Tips to Deal with Chlorine, Disinfection By-products, Fluoride, and Chromium-6:

- **Check your water supply by looking at the EWG's Tap Water Database (see Resources section for Action Step 6).**
- **For use with baby formula, use a reverse osmosis filter if your water is fluoridated. Otherwise use fluoride-free bottled water.**
- **Shorter, cooler showers can reduce inhalation exposure. Vent with a fan or open a window.**
- **Shower filters can remove chlorine but currently do not completely remove chloramine. Whole house water filters remove chlorine, chloramine, and other contaminants (see Action Step 6).**

37. Mind Your Devices

Cell phones, cordless phones, tablets, laptops, routers, smart meters, and even baby monitors all emit electromagnetic fields

(EMFs). This manmade radiation surrounds us in a sea of invisible energy of various frequencies, which may have possible health effects. The common belief that EMFs have no biological effects if they do not cause tissue heating has been challenged by a growing number of independent scientists who are concerned about long-term exposure to low-level microwave and cell phone radiation. And in 2014, the WHO's International Agency for Research on Cancer classified cell phone radiation as a "possible carcinogen," particularly for brain tumors.

Studies of cell phone use suggest greater risk of glioma (a type of cancerous brain tumor) with longer hours of use, more years of use, starting use prior to age 20, and lower power. Because their brain tissues are more absorbent, their skulls are thinner, and their relative size is smaller, children absorb more radiation and therefore have an increased risk to radiofrequency radiation compared to adults. Over twenty countries advise precautionary policies for use of WiFi in school, yet WiFi use in the United States is rapidly increasing. In addition to being a possible carcinogen, a number of studies have linked EMFs to disturbances of cognitive function, melatonin production, sleep, immune system function, and sperm count and quality.

Current Federal Communications Commission (FCC) guidelines for radiofrequency radiation emissions are outdated, with the last review conducted in the mid-1990s prior to the near universal use of cell phones and WiFi today. Other countries, however, are creating new policies to address these potential health risks, particularly for children. The European Parliament recommended that WiFi be removed from schools, daycares, retirement centers, and hospitals. Germany, Finland, the United Kingdom, and Russia have measures to protect children from EMFs. In 2015, France passed a law to limit exposure to EMFs including the ban of wireless devices in facilities that care for children under age three, very limited WiFi use in primary schools, safety warnings on advertisements, and clear signage for WiFi networks in public places. Some parts of India have also prohibited cell towers in certain areas and have dismantled thousands of cell towers.

In addition to potential health risks, it is estimated that approximately 2 to 10 percent of the population has electrosensitivity. People with electrosensitivity can exhibit a wide range of symptoms including pain, headaches, brain fog, sleep issues, low energy levels, and rashes in the presence of electromagnetic radiation. It often develops after a sudden excessive exposure to radiofrequency or electricity. Some can become very disabled and others may be unaware of the link between their EMF exposure and their symptoms. Often those sensitive to EMFs have an elevated total toxic load so reducing all types of toxic exposures and supporting detoxification can help.

The fact is that wireless technologies have not been around long enough or studied well enough to know if they definitively are harmful or not. In this case, I would use the precautionary principle and minimize unnecessary exposure when possible. You don't need to go completely off the grid to reduce your exposure. Start by dedicating at least one room in the house as a "safe haven" from EMF exposure, such as the bedroom. Unplug and disable all electronic and digital equipment in the room—at the very least, avoid having things plugged in near the bed. Some turn off the circuit breaker to the bedroom at night, and in Europe there are often switches to do so already built in. Put your cell phone and other devices on airplane mode, or better still, turn them off or keep them in another room.

Tips to Protect Yourself from EMFs:
- **Turn your phone, tablet, and computer off or put it into airplane mode (WiFi and Bluetooth off) when not in use.**
- **Keep your phone out of your bra and away from your pelvis, preferably away from your body. Keep your laptop off your lap.**

- Avoid using your device when the signal is weak. If service is poor, the phone boosts power to try to connect, potentially increasing exposures.
- Radiofrequency (RF) reflects from metal, producing radiation hot spots, so avoid using devices in cars, airplanes, trains, and elevators. In addition, when you are moving the continuous cell tower reconnections may increase RF exposure.
- Use an earpiece (corded or airtube style are the most protective) or speaker mode with your cell or wireless phone. Since radiation falls off rapidly with distance, the further away from your body, the better.
- Use wired (Ethernet) connections instead of wireless when possible.
- Use an automatic timer to turn your WiFi router off at night or turn it off manually.
- Consider replacing wireless devices like your mouse, keyboard, printer, speakers, and game consoles with wired ones. Most WiFi-enabled devices can be hardwired.
- Forward cell phone calls to a home landline to decrease cell phone use. At home, use a corded telephone or ECO-DECT cordless phone that only emits radiation when receiving and sending a call instead of continuously with a standard DECT cordless.
- A few products are available to shield from EMFs including RF-proof paint, shielding fabric, and cell phone and tablet covers. Be aware that using fabrics or other reflecting material may wear out some equipment faster and may also reflect the radiation so consulting with a building biologist may be important (see Resources section).
- Try to minimize your use of a transmitting device when your children are near. Turn WiFi and

Bluetooth off when children use the device if possible. Remove all wireless and screen devices from children's bedrooms.

- If you think you have electromagnetic hypersensitivity symptoms, keep a diary of your exposures and when your symptoms appear, and check for correlation. Discuss this with your doctor or healthcare provider.

- Consider consulting a professional EMF remediation expert. The Institute for Building Biology and Ecology can be a useful resource.

- Campaign with other parents to use hardwired networks in schools to provide Internet access. If unable or unwilling, request that WiFi be turned off when not in use. Educate children to use wireless technology safely.

- Let your elected officials know about your concerns and ask them to adopt policies to make wireless technology safer. Encourage them to fund education and research on electromagnetic radiation and health through a small fee attached to cell phone plans.

- Take a screen-free week to disconnect from devices and reconnect with life.

38. The Nanny State Against Toxic Toys

Unfortunately, no entity currently exists which ensures that the toys being sold in the United States are not toxic to our children. From endocrine-disrupting phthalates in plastics to lead paint and jewelry, you, as the parent, need to be the protector of your children's health. This is particularly important for young children as they often put toys in their mouths.

Top contaminants to avoid include lead on painted items and in play makeup, cadmium and lead in play jewelry, and phthalates in soft plastics (teethers, rubber duckies, and lunch boxes).

Choosing Safer Toys and Children's Products:

- **Buy toys from companies that let you know what the product is made out of.**
- **Look for products made from natural materials.**
  - For wood, choose unfinished or those with nontoxic paints and finishes.
  - Choose toys made from bioplastic (corn), natural rubber, and plant-based colorants to avoid harmful plastics and phthalates.
  - For plush toys, choose those made from hemp, organic cotton, and wool and colored with nontoxic dyes to avoid flame retardants, dyes, and foam filling.
- **If purchasing toys which have been painted, check where it was manufactured.** Toys made in China or India may contain lead paint. Avoid antique toys (pre-1978) as lead paint was commonly in use in the United States prior to that time.
- **Keep children from chewing or otherwise mouthing jewelry which may contain lead and cadmium.**
- **Avoid PVC (Plastic #3 or "V") and vinyl.** Look for phthalate-free toys. Avoid soft plastic toys made before 2009 in the United States or 2006 in Europe as they likely contain higher levels of phthalates.
- **Do not give children plastic teethers. Choose pacifiers made from clear silicone.**
- **For art supplies:**
  - Choose low-odor products like pens and markers and avoid anything with a warning label.
  - Choose soybean- or beeswax-based crayons and no-dust chalk.
  - Watercolor and water-based tempura paints are good choices as they typically have low or no volatile compounds.
  - Avoid polymer clays as they are made of PVCs softened with phthalates.

39. Keep Your Floors Clean

A 2015 study found that forty-five potentially toxic chemicals associated with health hazards such as cancer, endocrine and hormone disruption, and reproductive toxicity were commonly found in household dust. These included phthalates, environmental phenols, flame retardants, fragrances, and fluorinated chemicals. Household dust on your carpets and floors may also be a source of exposure for pesticide residues, lead dust, and VOCs.

Carpet

All carpets, whether synthetic or natural, gather and hold a large quantity of household dust and therefore can also hold a large quantity of toxic chemicals. So be sure to vacuum regularly with a HEPA filter to remove dust instead of a regular vacuum, which can disperse fine dusts back into the air. But what about the carpets themselves?

Synthetic carpets are made from petroleum by-products such as polypropylene, nylon, and acrylic and can contain dozens of toxic chemicals including carcinogens and solvents such as benzene, formaldehyde, and styrene. Carpets are also commonly treated with toxic flame retardants and stain protectors. The EPA considers synthetic carpet to be a major contributor of VOCs to indoor air pollution. The largest release of VOCs from new carpeting occurs in the first seventy-two hours after installation. However, low levels can continue to be emitted for years. Although natural, wool carpet can often contain pesticides to mothproof the wool so look for 100 percent organic options. In addition, carpet backing for synthetic and natural carpets may be made from vinyl, polypropylene, or synthetic latex; padding can contain PVC or urethane; and the adhesives used can also be full of VOCs.

Better options include natural fiber carpet with jute backings that have not been treated with pesticides or other chemicals. Wool is naturally flame and stain resistant. Hemp is more resistant to mold and mildew and may be a good choice for kitchens and bathrooms. Other fibers such as sisal, sea grass, jute, and coir (coconut-husk fiber) are becoming more widely available. Another option made from corn leaves and stalks is washable and compostable.

Other Flooring

Avoid synthetic flooring such as that made from vinyl (PVC), which can emit toxic gasses and comes from a toxic supply chain. Instead, choose natural and untreated materials: natural or "true" linoleum, untreated hardwood, bamboo, cork, ceramic tile, marble, stone, slate, or concrete. When installing new flooring, use low-VOC glues to avoid solvents such as toluene and benzene and choose finishes that are also low-VOC or go untreated. Wet mop frequently to decrease dust accumulation.

Never-Ending Hazards of PVC

Polyvinyl chloride (PVC) is used in a variety of products including vinyl flooring, wall coverings, countertops, miniblinds, window frames, shower curtains, pipes, ducts, raincoats, lunch boxes, art supplies, backpacks, toys, shoes, and food and beverage packaging. Although most people are aware that plastics are an environmental problem, the hazards of PVC go way beyond that of other plastics. Alternatives are available for almost every use, so why is it still being used?

This material is toxic throughout its life cycle. PVC is made from chlorine gas, an industrial by-product that is also a poison outlawed as a chemical weapon after World War I. Chlorine is combined with ethylene from natural gas to make ethylene chloride, which is a human carcinogen and contaminates water supplies. Ethylene chloride is then used to make vinyl chloride, also a potent human carcinogen which is explosively flammable and is transported via train to

PVC plants (a 2012 train derailment in New Jersey released thousands of pounds of this toxin into the air) where it is combined with other polymers such as vinyl acetate (an explosive carcinogen). The production of PVC releases dioxin, a carcinogen and hormone disruptor that is persistent in the environment. PVC needs a number of additives to make it useable including lead, cadmium, organotins, phthalates, and fire retardants, which can separate from the PVC and also contaminate your home. PVC products do not biodegrade, leaching phthalates and heavy metals when landfilled. Recycling is not easily accomplished and would release toxic substances. Burning of PVC creates dioxin and generates black, choking smoke. Exposure to PVC has also been linked to asthma and lung problems. In 2016 an explosion and subsequent fire at a PVC plant in Louisiana released toxic pollutants into the surrounding community and led to a closure of a 45-mile section of the Mississippi River.

Many manufacturers are making PVC-free products such as shower curtains, but it is still widely in use. Avoid plastic #3, which is PVC. Unfortunately, you must be aware of each product and perform your due diligence if you want to completely eliminate this toxic substance from your life. The Resources section has some suggestions on how to find PVC-free toys, school supplies, and building materials.

Tips to Keep Your Floors Clean:
- **Use a HEPA vacuum on carpets and wet mop other flooring regularly.**
- **Remove shoes before coming indoors.**
- **Place natural doormats at each entrance.**
- **Choose nontoxic or natural flooring and ensure that backing, padding, glues, and any finishes used are also nontoxic.**

40. Don't Live in a Moldy Home

Just because you don't see molds in your house doesn't mean you don't have them. They can be hiding in drywall, insulation, and plywood, which they thrive on. Most people who live or work in buildings with toxic mold issues are totally unaware that there is any problem. Even when mold is visible, it may appear like a smear of dirt on the wall leading many people to miss it. It often cannot be smelled either.

Molds are known to play a role in asthma, allergies, sinus, and lung problems. They have also been associated with many other health conditions including skin rashes, immune compromise, chronic fatigue, gastrointestinal complaints, chronic pain, and neurological problems. Those who are sick may have no idea that their issue stems from toxic mold.

According to the EPA, all molds have the potential to affect health. They are classified into three groups: allergenic molds, pathogenic molds, which can cause an infection in immune compromised people, and toxigenic, or toxic molds which produce harmful mycotoxins. Molds produce a number of substances that can affect your health such as VOCs, respiratory inhalants, and mycotoxins.

Mycotoxins are toxins that are present on spores and small fragments of mold released into the air. Even spores that are no longer able to reproduce can still harm your health due to these mycotoxins. Mycotoxins are easily absorbed through skin, airways, and intestinal lining and can interfere with RNA synthesis and potentially cause DNA damage. Trichothecenes are a particularly hazardous type of mycotoxin produced by a variety of molds including *Stachybotrys*, otherwise known as black mold.

In genetically susceptible people (certain HLA-gene haplotypes), biotoxins such as mycotoxins are not cleared easily from the body. This explains why the effects of toxicity may be different in each person, why some people in the same household may not appear to be affected, and why some people are able to live in their mold-infested home until an event tips them over and they become sensitized to the mold toxins. If you suspect that you have an illness triggered by mold and mold toxins, seek the help of a practitioner who has experience in biotoxin or mold-related illnesses.

Our homes are an optimal environment for molds to grow and mold spores are everywhere. All that they need to grow is oxygen, the optimal temperature, a food source (the building materials in our homes—they just love drywall), plus a water source. When a leak occurs, it only takes twenty-four to forty-eight hours for mold to start growing. It doesn't even have to be a big leak—it can be just a slow drip. When mold is found, however, it is not enough to just fix the leak and dry out the area. The mold can remain toxic even after it no longer has access to water and stops growing. In fact, stopping the source of water can potentially make a toxic mold problem even worse, since dried-up colonies tend to release more spores into the air than live colonies. Because of the way that mold spores spread, it can travel to many areas of the home. Therefore, finding all the places where mold is growing and addressing it properly is important, not just dealing with the obvious mold growing in the open. To keep the toxins contained and prevent further spread of mold spores, a professional remediation company using hazardous materials protocols is recommended. Although expensive, this is the only way to safely remove toxic mold and avoid further spread of spores which can create further problems.

Most toxic mold problems that make people sick occur in three places: inside drywall, inside wall or attic insulation, and inside HVAC systems. But toxic mold may be hidden in other places such as inside crawl spaces or behind wallpaper, fake paneling, or shower enclosures. The source of water can come from plumbing leaks as well as condensation between walls, in the HVAC system, or from portable air conditioners; even very dry climates with low humidity may have toxic mold growth in these areas.

Tests for Mold

There is currently no singular test that can assess the level of mold in a home with absolute certainty when mold is not visible and cultured, therefore several methods may be used. If you have visible mold which is then sent for culture and comes back positive, however, that is pretty darn certain.

Urine testing: Fifteen mycotoxins associated with the most common molds found in water-damaged buildings (trichothecenes, ochratoxin, aflatoxin, and gliotoxin derivative) are measurable in morning urine by RealTime Labs for about $699. Great Plains Lab released a urine mycotoxin test for $299 in September 2017 that screens for seven different mycotoxins from four species of mold including those found in water-damaged buildings as well as mold-contaminated foods. A positive test indicates recent exposure. You then want to determine where the exposure is coming from and consider further testing. However, this test is not covered by insurance.

Environmental Relative Moldiness Index (ERMI): Developed by the EPA, this looks for the genetic markers of thirty-six different mold species in a dust sample which may be sampled by wipes or vacuum. The report provides a score that evaluates the likelihood of presence of toxic molds. Although this is a test most recommended by mold specialists, it may miss hidden mold problems. The cost is around $200 to $300.

HERTSMI-2: Similar to ERMI, except that it looks for the presence of only five particularly dangerous species of mold: *Aspergillus penicilloides, Aspergillus versicolor, Chaetomium globosum, Stachybotrys chartarum*, and *Wallemia sebi*. The cost is lower than ERMI.

Air testing: This test looks for the presence of mold spores in the air at a particular moment in time to evaluate the amount of mold present, the types of mold present, and how indoor samples compare with outdoor samples. Since it looks at whole spores instead of genetic material, it may miss certain species of mold such as *Stachybotrys*, which releases spores in waves and also has heavy spores that rapidly fall to the ground and then break up into fragments which are then carried to other locations. This type of testing, however, may be most helpful for allergies and asthma. These tests are usually done by indoor air quality professionals and may cost $1,000 or more.

Air sampling with DNA analysis: This is now becoming available and is an improvement on traditional air sampling; however, it does not appear to be in wide use as yet.

Petri dish test: Culture plates are placed in several areas around the house as well as outside. Some molds do not grow well on culture plates and therefore this is not a very reliable test.

Hire a professional: The Indoor Air Quality Association can be a good starting place to search for mold inspectors. Ask for their qualifications and certifications and if they have any building science training or are industrial hygienists, which may be a plus.

Tips to Reduce Exposure to Toxic Mold:

- **Do not use carpeting in wet areas such as the bathroom or basement, which provides food for mold to grow on.**
- **Plumbing leaks are one of the leading causes of mold growth. Check under kitchen and bathroom sinks, around water heaters, and behind washing machines and dishwashers. Inspect caulking around shower and tub areas and make sure that it is intact.**
- **Identify and address any leaks which caused water damage within forty-eight hours.**

- If you see visible mold, do not touch or cut into the area without properly sealing the area off to prevent spread of mold spores throughout the rest of your home. Contact a mold remediation specialist.
- Use a HEPA room air filter regularly and change its location in the room on a daily basis to clean the whole area.
- Consider testing to assess possible exposure to toxic mold. Work with a health professional familiar with biotoxins or mold-related illnesses if you believe you have been affected.
- If you have toxic mold in your home:
  - Use a professional mold remediation service to protect from further contamination. Often they have to wear hazmat suits.
  - Mold spores become embedded within any porous items including books, carpets, photos, paper, and upholstered material, which need to be replaced.
  - If clothing smells moldy or sweet and pungent it likely cannot be salvaged. Clothing may be cleaned if not contaminated.
  - Nonporous items like wood, glass, plastic, and metal can be cleaned.
  - The level of cleaning you need depends on your genetic susceptibility for mold toxin illness: there are two types that require more diligence. A health professional trained in this area can help you determine this.
  - Lipoic acid, glutathione, and other nutrients can help protect against, or reverse the adverse effects of, mycotoxins.

41. Get the Lead Out and Don't Lick Your Deck

Heavy metal isn't just a type of music: these natural elements have been used by humans for thousands of years and also have been associated with adverse health effects. Exposure to heavy metals can come from a variety of sources: airborne sources, carbonated beverages in aluminum cans, cooking utensils, dental amalgams, food additives, food contaminants, glass, lead building materials, lead plumbing, products containing lead, tap water, vaccine additives, and outdoor wood structures. I have discussed mercury in seafood and lead in water elsewhere, but let's also take a look at a few other common contaminants: arsenic, cadmium, and aluminum.

Arsenic

Arsenic is found naturally in groundwater and exposure to arsenic is mainly via drinking water and food supply. It is a known poison, disrupts mitochondria, and is known to cause cancer and diabetes. In 2001, the National Academy of Sciences reported that arsenic causes cancer in humans "at doses that are close to the drinking-water concentrations that occur in the United States." Long-term exposure to arsenic in drinking water is mainly related to increased risks of skin cancer but also some other cancers, as well as other skin lesions such as hyperkeratosis and pigmentation changes. Arsenic is also in the food supply with 80 percent of dietary arsenic intake from meat, fish, and poultry because arsenic is in pesticides, herbicides, and fungicides used in animal feed and production. Arsenic has made the news in recent years, having been found in some wines, rice, and chicken. Arsenic is also released in environmental tobacco smoke. At low levels, arsenic has been associated with high blood pressure in pregnant mothers.

A less obvious source of arsenic may be in your backyard. If you have a wood deck, picnic table, or playground set made before 2005, chances are it contains arsenic as 90 percent of outdoor wooden structures in the United States are made of pressure treated wood. Usually tinted green, pressure-treated wood is treated with chromium, copper, and arsenic (CCA) to preserve it. Arsenic from this wood has been found to leach out and can be absorbed through the skin and contaminate the soil. If you have CCA-treated wood in your yard, replace it if you can. Do not burn the wood as it will release toxic arsenic into the air. Do not use it as compost or near edible plants. Instead, treat it as the hazardous waste that it is and contact your local sanitation department for information on how to dispose of it.

If you cannot get rid of arsenic-treated wood or if you visit a community park that still has these structures, definitely do not eat off of it! Make sure you and your children wash your hands after touching it, especially before eating. Keep shoes outdoors on a doormat before going indoors from a deck or after playing on a wood structure. Sealing the wood may help, although it is not known to what extent, and it should be resealed at least every six months.

Cadmium

Cadmium is found in high concentrations in cigarette smoke and at lower levels in our food supply. It disrupts mitochondria, causes cancer and kidney damage, acts as a xenoestrogen, and increases the risk of osteoporosis. Cadmium compounds are currently mainly used in rechargeable nickel-cadmium batteries. It is also used in metal plating, plastics, and textile manufacturing. Airborne emissions have increased dramatically during the twentieth century, presumably because cadmium-containing products are rarely recycled but often dumped together with household waste. Make sure to take your rechargeable cadmium batteries to the proper disposal location. Cadmium occurs naturally in many foods because it is present in soil and water. Some of the foods higher in cadmium include potatoes, sunflower seeds, peanuts, fish, shellfish, and soy products, including tofu. Cadmium also accumulates in leafy vegetables such as spinach and other plants as a result of cadmium-contaminated fertilizer, which is also used often on grass.

Aluminum

Aluminum is ubiquitous in the environment, accumulates in the body, and has been linked to a number of different health issues including neurologic and immunologic problems. Common sources include aluminum-contaminated water, aluminum cookware (especially if water is fluoridated), aluminum foil, and aluminum-containing antiperspirants and medications (such as antacids). Some foods, like baking powder and processed cheeses, have higher than natural levels of aluminum because they contain aluminum-based food additives. Aluminum is also the most commonly used vaccine adjuvant—a substance used to trigger an immune response.

Mercury

Mercury is a known health hazard with three main types causing different effects including fatigue. Methylmercury is a known neurotoxin and is widespread in our environment and ends up in our food chain. Elemental (metallic) mercury is an issue when mercury is spilled and vapors are inhaled and is found in compact fluorescent light (CFL) bulbs, old mercury thermometers, and dental amalgams. Inorganic mercury is produced from elemental mercury through the process of oxidation and is the most common form in drinking water. This type is used in the chemical industry and is found in batteries. Other mercury compounds like ethylmercury are found in products such as thimerosal, which is used in multi-dose flu vaccines as a preservative.

The single largest source of mercury in our environment is in the air from coal-burning power plants. The airborne mercury eventually settles into bodies of water like lakes, streams, rivers, and coastal waters. In the water, elemental mercury is transformed to methylmercury by microorganisms and then is eaten by and accumulated in fish and shellfish. Fish advisories are in effect in many states as there is such widespread contamination of waterbodies with mercury (see Action Step

5 for details on safer fish). In addition, pregnant women are advised to limit consumption of certain fish that tend to be higher in mercury—each year 630,000 children are born at risk for neurodevelopmental problems due to prenatal mercury exposure. Mercury crosses the blood-brain barrier and placenta and is distributed to all tissues but targets the brain, kidneys, and liver. Mercury is excreted predominantly in the feces (90 percent) and some through sweat and urine. It can be reabsorbed in the colon, so those with chronic constipation are at increased risk of recycling mercury back into their system. It is estimated that 5 percent is excreted in breast milk.

Another avenue of exposure to mercury is through dental amalgams, which are silver-colored fillings made from a combination of liquid mercury and other metals. Although the FDA considers these to be safe for adults and children over the age of six, it is also acknowledged that about 1 microgram of mercury can be released from each filling each day as mercury vapor. The amount of mercury released increases with heat and trauma, including chewing hot foods and drinking hot coffee or other hot beverages. Mercury vapors are also released when amalgam fillings are placed or removed from teeth. Improper management of dental amalgam waste contributes to environmental contamination of land, air, and water and dental offices are the single largest source of mercury at sewage treatment plants. There are a number of alternative restorative materials which can be used for fillings instead of mercury.

Lead

Lead can be found throughout our environment and can affect almost every organ in the body with particular harm for brain and nervous system development in young children. It is estimated that one million children (4.4 percent of all preschoolers) have blood lead at levels known to affect intelligence, cause learning disabilities, and cause permanent brain and nervous system damage. Those who have osteoporosis are also at increased risk of elevated blood lead levels as lead is released during bone loss.

Exposure comes from a variety of products found in and around our homes including use of lead-based paint (prior to 1978), leaded gasoline (fully phased out in the United States in 1996, but present in soil near roadways), ceramics (including food containers), pipes, solder, batteries, cosmetics, candy from Mexico, vinyl mini-blinds, boxed wines, and imported traditional Chinese and Ayurvedic herbal remedies. Lead has also been found in children's toys and jewelry. Lead is in the air from ore and metals processing and leaded airplane fuel and can contribute to the amount of lead in soil, dust, and water. Lead in soil can be an exposure route for young children, can contribute to lead dust in the home as it is tracked in from outdoors, and can be taken up by plants grown on the soil, contaminating food and herbal remedies. As we have recently learned from the Flint, Michigan, tragedy that has now called attention to the 5,300 plus cities that have lead violations in the water, corrosion from old pipes combined with acidic water is a huge problem as well.

Tips to Reduce Heavy Metal Exposure:
- **Avoid tracking dust inside by taking shoes off indoors and using doormats at each entrance. Use HEPA air filters and vacuums, and clean floors and dust frequently.**
- **Wash hands with soap and water after being outdoors, especially before eating.**
- **Don't smoke cigarettes (see Action Step 24 on tips to quit).**
- **Check your water quality. If needed, get a water filter to remove contaminants (see Action Steps 6 and 36).**
- **Avoid CCA treated (green-tinted) pressurized wood and remove it from your home area if possible, checking with your local sanitation department for proper**

disposal. If it is in a public park, petition to have it removed and properly disposed of.

- Limit or avoid foods that have high levels of mercury, arsenic, cadmium, aluminum, and lead, including large fish and fish from the Great Lakes, soy/tofu, certain wines, aluminum containing baking powder, processed cheese, candy from Mexico, and certain types of rice (jasmine and basmati rice tend to have less arsenic than brown rice and rice from California and Southeast Asia have less arsenic than rice grown in other parts of the United States). Rinse rice well and cook in extra water.
- Use non-aluminum cookware.
- Dispose of CFL bulbs, old mercury thermometers, and batteries properly.
- Choose alternative fillings rather than silver amalgams. If silver amalgams need to be removed, make sure your dentist follows International Academy of Oral Medicine and Toxicology (IAOMT) guidelines on safe removal (see Resources).
- Check safecosmetics.org or EWG's Skin Deep database to be sure your cosmetics are lead-free.
- Be careful of possible lead in toys especially imported toys, antique toys, and toy jewelry. The most harm comes if the child chews or otherwise mouths the toy or jewelry.
- Avoid using containers, cookware, or tableware to store or cook foods or liquids that are not shown to be lead free, particularly glazed ceramic.
- Purchase herbal remedies from a reliable source that tests each batch for heavy metal contamination which can come from the soil.
- If you live in a pre-1978 home, you may have lead paint on your walls and woodwork. Contact your

local government authority about testing for lead
dust in your carpet.

- Lead pipes were used in houses built before the
1920s and lead solder was used to join copper piping
between the 1950s and the 1980s. Run cold water for
two to five minutes before using to flush the pipes
of standing water before use and consider testing
your water for lead and other contaminants.

- Avoid vinyl mini-blinds, boxed wines with vinyl
pouches, and metal wicked candles which may be
contaminated by lead.

42. What's in the Garage?

Attached garages are wonderfully convenient but may also
contribute to toxicity in your home. In fact, the largest
source of poor indoor air quality according to the EPA is an
attached garage, mostly due to car emissions. When our cars
are running in the garage, they emit fumes including carbon monoxide, benzene, polycyclic aromatic hydrocarbons,
and particulate matter, which can all cause negative health
effects. Then when we shut the exterior garage door, those
toxins are trapped in the garage and can enter the home.
If you must have an attached garage, don't idle your engine
in the garage, and keep the exterior garage door open for a
few minutes to vent after parking. Garage ventilation systems
may also be installed.

Another reason why garages (and storage sheds) can be
hazardous is that they can become storage facilities for dangerous chemicals we use for home, garden, and auto maintenance. Paints, thinners, glues and adhesives, insect sprays,
weed killers, cleaners, antifreeze, motor oil, swimming pool
chemicals—many of these contain chemicals that can become
volatile and spread into the air. A garage ventilation system
would also help the air in this case, but reducing these toxic
products can help to avoid toxic exposures in general. In other

sections of this book, I have described less toxic alternatives to many of these products.

Tips to Detoxify Your Garage:

- **Park outside or ventilate the garage for a few minutes after parking. Do not idle your engine in the garage.**
- **Keep dangerous products stored out of children's reach.**
- **Always ventilate when using toxic products or use them outdoors.**
- **Choose less toxic products and dispose of old toxic products properly by finding out how to dispose of household hazardous waste in your community.**

43. Rethink Your Pest Control

Pesticides are designed to kill, and not surprisingly they can also be dangerous to people, pets, and other wildlife. The home and garden are two areas where people are exposed to pest-control products that contain active pesticides as well as "inert" ingredients that may actually be toxic to humans such as formaldehyde, benzene, and aniline. Due to trade secrecy laws, however, those "inert" ingredients do not have to be listed on the product label, so you may be exposed to harmful chemicals without knowing it.

The category of organochlorine pesticides includes more than 15,000 chemicals. They can cause damage to the endocrine, immune, and detoxification systems and are sometimes given to animals to induce disease to be studied. People and pets may be at more risk from using these chemical pesticides than from the insects they are trying to control. Pesticides are especially hazardous to children, who spend more time closer to the ground where these chemicals are often applied. Kids are also less resilient to these toxic chemicals than adults, and their developing brains are more susceptible to neurological problems and learning disabilities caused by exposure. Of all the cases of pesticide poisoning in the United States, half of them are in kids under six. In addition, pesticides are a key factor in explaining honey bee population declines; bees are important for one-third of human food production, and 90 percent of wild plants are dependent on pollination.

A basic principle of Integrated Pest Management (IPM) is to try preventive and nontoxic alternatives as a first line defense against pests and use toxic pesticides as a last resort. Many effective options exist that do not utilize pesticides. Starting with quality soil can help build healthy and insect-resistant plants. Some plants may also attract beneficial insects and birds to control harmful insect populations and some may be more resistant to pests naturally. To combat pests like aphids, caterpillars, and moths, we release ladybugs and praying mantises into the garden. Other beneficial insects include: decollate snails, which get rid of harmful snails and do not damage vegetation; predatory nematodes, which are effective against over 250 species of insects that have a soil-dwelling stage such as Japanese beetles and white grubs; and green lacewings, which eat many small insects including aphids and caterpillars. In addition, practices such as crop rotation can strengthen the plants and the surrounding environment. Other environmentally friendly methods include using pheromone-based insect traps and bio-mimicry deterrents. IPM can be a low-cost, environmentally friendly solution.

The first line of defense with IPM is preventing pests from entering your home. Repair ripped windows and door screens, seal bathroom and kitchen cracks with silicone caulk, and plug openings throughout the home that are larger than ¼ inch wide with cement, steel wool, or other metals. The next step is to deny pests shelter, food, and water. If you have holes in your floorboards, replace them before ants or termites can infest the rotting wood. Recycle old newspapers before rodents shred them and use the scraps to build their nests. Don't leave food out, mop up spills, sweep and vacuum regularly, wash dishes, take out the garbage, and keep garbage cans clean of food residue. Fix any leaks promptly.

If you must use pesticides, use these chemicals sparingly, with spot treatments limited to affected areas instead of spraying the whole house. Use pesticides with the lowest toxicity (those labeled IV on a scale of I to IV). Avoid chemicals that are known to be carcinogens, neurotoxins, and endocrine disrupters. If you need a professional exterminator, those certified by programs such as EcoWise, GreenPro, and Green Shield use IPM techniques.

Bee Mindful of Pesticide Use

A quote attributed to Albert Einstein says, "If the bee disappears from the surface of the Earth, man would have no more than four years to live. No more bees, no more pollination … no more men!" Bees make up about one-fifth of the world's pollinators, along with butterflies and certain flies, beetles, butterflies, birds, bats, and reptiles. These pollinators are responsible for an about one-third of the food that we eat. In recent years, honeybees have been decimated by Colony Collapse Disorder, and in 2015, American beekeepers lost an estimated 42 percent of their hives.

Although many factors likely are contributing to the declining bee population, studies suggest that a relatively new class of pesticides called neonicotinoids (neonics), which are among the most widely used in the world, are both indirectly and directly harming bees. This has prompted reevaluation by the EPA and regulation in Canada and the EU (France has a total ban and the EU has had a temporary ban since 2013). As of this writing, Maryland has become the first state to pass restrictions on the use of neonicotinoids and Ortho, a leading brand of home and garden pest-control products, announced it will stop using neonicotinoids in their products. In the meantime, watch out for these pesticides in products: imidacloprid, clothianidin, thiamethoxam, dinotefuran, and acetamiprid. A recent study found that 75 percent of honey samples tested worldwide between 2012 and 2016 contained neonics and nearly half were at levels that exceeded the minimum level to cause "marked detrimental effects" in pollinators. Neonics also pose a risk to frogs, common birds, fish, and earthworms.

Try These Nontoxic Methods to Combat Specific Pests:

Ants:

- **Keep ants away by spraying with a mixture of half vinegar and half water. Or mix 1 cup of water with 2 teaspoons of essential peppermint oil and spray wherever the ants are coming in.**
- **Sprinkle diatomaceous earth (wear a mask when doing so to avoid inhaling particles), which is harmful to the ants when eaten but not to humans or pets. This natural mineral is the fossilized skeletal remains of microscopic organisms and can be used against fleas, cockroaches, and slugs as well.**
- **Dust cracks and crevices with boric acid powder, which will slowly poison crawling insects but is less toxic to humans than pesticides. Also consider scrubbing affected areas with insecticidal or fatty-acid soaps, which are safe for people unless accidentally ingested. Keep kids and pets away from these solutions.**

Cockroaches:

- **Mix equal parts baking soda and powdered sugar and spread where cockroaches congregate. Repeat every one to two weeks until they are gone.**

- An alternative is to mix boric acid powder with sugar in a 2:1 ratio and sprinkle it in crevices for roaches and ants.

Snails and Slugs:
- Create a barrier made of copper wire or tape.
- Sprinkle diatomaceous earth or other gritty substances like crushed eggshells, or spread coffee grounds or iron phosphate baits.

Fleas:
- Use products for your pets that contain natural repellents such as pennyroyal or eucalyptus oil.

Head Lice

About six to twelve million children ages three to eleven get head lice each year in the United States. Eager to eliminate these infestations, many reach for over-the-counter remedies that contain harsh pesticides. Even worse, head lice have now become mostly resistant to these treatments so you may be using these toxic products without any benefit. Other nontoxic remedies do exist, including smothering them by saturating the scalp and hair with mayonnaise or oil and then leaving it to sit for at least two hours while covered with a plastic bag or shower cap. Then use a nit comb to remove all eggs that remain on the hair shaft followed by shampoo to remove the oil. Certain essential oils such as tea tree and neem are also effective against lice. Because this is such an issue, there is a growing industry of businesses specializing in pesticide-free lice treatment and many of them go to the clients' home.

---

44. Weed by Hand, Not Poison

Weeds can be the bane of existence for many gardeners who may reach for chemical weed killers to easily handle dandelions and the like. But similar to pesticides, these formulations are made from harmful chemicals like 2,4-dichlorophenoxyacetic acid (2,4-D) and glyphosate (Roundup) as well as "inert" ingredients that may also cause harm to humans and other creatures. In addition to contamination of our immediate environment, these chemicals also end up in our water supply.

2,4-D has been linked to cancer, kidney, and liver damage, reproductive toxicity, endocrine disruption, and nervous system damage. Many 2,4-D products also contain dioxins, which are carcinogenic, affect fertility and hormones, and cause miscarriage and birth defects. This compound has been found to accumulate in house dust even days after spraying outside. Glyphosate is one of the most widely used weed killers and is patented as an antibiotic and a chelating agent—binding to many essential nutrients. It has been linked to disruption of hormonal systems, reduction of beneficial gut bacteria, DNA damage, developmental and reproductive toxicity, birth defects, cancer, and neurotoxicity. The product Roundup uses glyphosate as well as an "inert" ingredient called polyethoxylated tallow amine (POEA). Studies have shown that this supposedly "inert" component actually caused more damage to human embryonic, placental, and umbilical cord cells than glyphosate alone. A newer product called Enlist Duo combines 2,4-D and Roundup and is sprayed on GMO crops Enlist corn and Enlist soy. 2,4-D is persistent and pervasive in the environment. Depending on the formulation, it can drift through the air from the fields where it is sprayed or be tracked inside homes and schools by pets or children. 2,4-D has already been detected in groundwater, surface water, and drinking water, and in 2012 it was found in more than 90 percent of samples taken from agricultural catchments bordering the Great Barrier Reef. This substance is not only toxic for many fish but also can poison small mammals, including dogs who can ingest it while eating grass treated with 2,4-D.

Tips to Eliminate Weeds without Toxic Herbicides:

- Plant native species to compete with weeds.
- Mulch. Spread about one inch of shredded fall leaves, straw, or clippings from an herbicide-free lawn or use bark mulch.
- Spray weeds with vinegar. The vinegar will kill almost all plants, so avoid spraying plants you want to keep.
- Sprays work best when the weeds are dry and it is sunny. They are less effective on a cool, cloudy, or wet day.
- Herbicidal soap sprays kill weeds by smothering them with a soap bubble-like film.
- If the soil is moist, pull weeds by hand. Be sure to remove roots to prevent re-sprouting.
- Ask your local government to follow suit of other municipalities and stop spraying for roadside weed control and particularly to restrict use at childcare facilities, schools, and playgrounds.

45. Skip the Lawn

It is only in the last century that lawns became a hallmark of American suburban life. And they have grown to account for eighty million home lawns and a $40 billion per year industry. It can take a lot of work requiring seed, fertilizer, an irrigation system, Weedwackers, herbicides, pesticides, mowers, mower maintenance, and of course water. And all of this effort to keep a green lawn can also be harmful to us and our environment.

More than two-thirds of America's home lawns are treated with chemical fertilizers or pesticides with more than sixty-seven million pounds of synthetic chemicals sprayed every year. As I mentioned in the last two sections, pesticides and herbicides are potential toxins that can be harmful to human health. And not only are we exposed to them outdoors, they also get tracked in and contaminate dust in our homes where they can persist. In addition to adverse human health effects, herbicides like 2,4-D have other negative downstream consequences. Since 2,4-D preserves grass but kills weeds like clover, which fixes nitrogen, soil becomes nitrogen-poor and cannot support plant life, necessitating use of synthetic nitrogen fertilizers. These fertilizers are water-soluble and end up in runoff after watering or rain. When that runoff ends up in a waterway, the nitrogen can create algae blooms that end up depleting oxygen from the river, lake, or bay. These areas become dead zones where plants and fish cannot survive. Because of this effect, nitrogen runoff is considered to be one of the worst problems for water quality. Pesticides, herbicides, and fungicides also contaminate the waterways.

Another reason why green lawns are bad for our environment is the amount of water used. The EPA estimated that the average American household uses about forty-eight gallons of water per day for lawns and gardens. Nationwide approximately nine billion gallons of water are used per day just for landscape irrigation! This is an incredible amount of water and at the very least we should utilize non-potable reclaimed water, which in the United States and some other countries is distributed in purple pipes.

For these reasons, I encourage you to switch from a green lawn to more native plants. Living in Southern California where we tend to struggle with water shortages, I have been impressed by how beautiful the alternatives can be. Many are turning to xeriscaping, which reduces or eliminates the need for supplemental irrigation. But if you are not ready to go all in, then I encourage you to at least "green" your lawn care to make it healthier for you, your family, and the environment. At the very least, leave your shoes at the front door so you are not tracking chemicals into your house and have your children wash their hands after playing on the lawn or a publicly maintained field.

How to Green Your Lawn Care:

- Switch from a green lawn to native plants and dry creek beds.
- Start with great soil. Have it tested to find out what you need to make it better.
- Plant clover with your grass, which competes with weeds and provides nitrogen in the soil, reducing the need for synthetic fertilizers.
- Leave your grass taller, which makes it more resistant to weeds and leave the clippings, which act as fertilizer. To be uber-green, use a push mower, which reduces pollutants and gives you a workout.
- Cut back watering to about once a week. Frequent watering leads to shallow roots.
- Use beneficial insects rather than pesticides.
- Weed by hand when soil is moist.

46. Compost to Create Black Gold

Several years ago, our neighbors wanted to know what we were doing to get such lush plants in our yard. The answer was compost—organic material that can be added to soil to help plants grow. Because it is so nutrient dense and provides so many other beneficial properties, gardeners consider it "black gold". In addition to providing nutrients, compost can increase water retention of soil, improve drought tolerance, prevent the growth of weeds, improve soil microorganisms, and reduce the need for fertilizers and chemicals.

Composting can help your backyard plants and also helps the environment by reducing the amount of food and yard waste going to landfills. The Natural Resources Defense Council (NRDC) reported that 40 percent of food in the United States goes uneaten (about 20 pounds per person each month!) and 97 percent of food waste ends up in landfills. According to the EPA, food waste is currently the single largest component of municipal solid waste going to landfills and incinerators. When food and yard waste are buried in a landfill and decompose without exposure to air, methane is produced—a greenhouse gas that is roughly twenty times more potent than carbon dioxide. To remedy this situation, some communities include curbside composting as part of their waste management services, but unfortunately this is not a universal practice. I must admit, I always felt a little guilty when I didn't get to my vegetables on time and needed to pitch them in the trash. But now if that happens I don't see it as a total waste but rather a renewable resource that is going to feed my garden. We have a compost crock in our kitchen where we collect food scraps regularly to take out to our compost pile.

While compost can be purchased, it is also easy to make your own compost at home. Composting requires just three basic ingredients: "green" materials such as fruit and vegetable scraps, eggshells, coffee grounds, and grass and plant clippings to provide nitrogen; "brown" materials such as dead leaves, shredded newspaper, straw, and finely chopped wood, branches, and twigs to provide carbon; and water, which provides moisture to help break down the organic matter.

To start your own backyard compost, select a dry, shady spot near a water source for your pile or bin. A bin helps contain your compost pile, makes it more attractive, and can be purchased or you can make your own. The bin should be at least three feet wide and three feet deep to provide enough space to mix or turn the ingredients. A cover or tarp is helpful to keep the compost moist. Your compost pile should have an equal amount of green and brown materials mixed together. Moisten with water as needed so that it has the consistency of a damp sponge, but do not overwater as this will lead to rotting. Add green and brown materials as they are available, burying fruit and vegetable waste under compost as you add it to your pile. Turn the compost pile about once a week to provide oxygen; this helps the materials decay faster and prevents foul odors. When the compost has become dark brown and crumbly it is ready to use in the garden. Depending on the conditions of your pile this can take from two months to more than a year.

Some items you **do not** want to put in your compost pile: meat, oil, fat, grease, dairy products, pet waste, diseased plant materials, pressure-treated or painted wood, and weeds that go to seed.

Tips to Turn Food and Yard Waste into "Black Gold":

- **Collect kitchen scraps in a compost crock to add to your outdoor compost pile.**
- **Purchase or build your own compost bin.**
- **Ask your waste management company if they will provide curbside composting to reduce food and yard waste contributions to landfills.**

47. Go Natural and Get Dirty

Currently half of the world lives in urban areas where they are not exposed to nature. Spending time in nature has been linked to improved mood (with increases in the "feel good" neurotransmitter serotonin), lower levels of depression and feelings of stress, and brain activity in areas responsible for empathy, emotional stability, and love. On the other hand, urban environments are associated with increases in fear and anxiety. Nature also may affect our immune function; a study at Tokyo's Nippon Medical School found that women who spent six hours in the woods over the course of two days had an increase in virus- and tumor-fighting white blood cells, which lasted at least seven days afterwards.

You don't have to travel to a nature preserve or live in the wild to experience nature. Even short exposures can have benefits. A 2010 study published in *Environmental Science and Technology* found that as little as five minutes in a natural setting, whether walking in a park or gardening in the backyard, improves mood, self-esteem, and motivation.

Some cultures embrace the healing benefits of nature therapy. In Japan, researchers studying "forest therapy," also called "forest bathing," have found that spending time in the woods creates measurable health benefits. It lowers levels of salivary cortisol, lowers blood pressure and pulse rate, and can enhance activity of natural killer (NK) cells, which are important immune system players that fight infection and cancer. Part of the positive effect may be attributed to inhalation of phytoncides, compounds in volatile oils given off by trees and other aromatic plants. In Norway, *friluftsliv* translates directly from Norwegian as "free air life" and is the concept that being outside is good for a human being's mind and spirit. It describes a way of life that is spent exploring and appreciating nature from walking in a natural area to sleeping outside to hiking. And there is a recent trend in "forest schools" for preschool and kindergarten, which have exploration in nature as a key element of their curriculum.

While actually being in nature is the ideal way to get the benefits of soil microbes, fresh air, phytoncides, and negative ion balance, merely looking at natural surroundings also has benefits. An early study by environmental psychologist Roger Ulrich showed that patients recovering from gallbladder surgery healed faster and with fewer complications when their room looked out on trees rather than a wall. In 1993, Ulrich and his colleagues also found that heart surgery patients in the intensive care unit who were given a water or tree scene to view were less anxious and needed less pain medication than those who were assigned a darker forest photograph, abstract art or no pictures at all. A Japanese study in 2005 showed that just gazing at forest scenery for twenty minutes reduced salivary cortisol (stress hormone) levels by 13.4 percent, bringing them down to lower-than-average concentrations among city dwellers. In 2010 researchers in Korea found that people who were shown pictures of scenic, natural landscapes had increased brain activity in areas associated with recall of pleasant memories as compared to people shown urban landscapes

Bring Nature into Your Life, Knowing that You are Part of Nature:

- Plant a garden, even if it is on your windowsill. Bring flowers or live plants into your home or office.
- Listen to birdsong—in nature or listen to a recording.
- Visit a park or botanical garden and sit or walk without checking your phone. Breathe in the air and notice the aroma of the plants.
- Watch the changing shapes of clouds or gaze at the stars and planets in the night sky.
- Observe a body of water—anything from a tabletop fountain to the crashing waves of an ocean.
- Stand in the sunlight for at least ten minutes, feeling the warmth of the sun's rays on your body.
- Walk barefoot on the earth, noticing how it feels on your feet.

Autobiography in 5 Short Chapters
by Portia Nelson

— act 1 —

I walk, down the street,
there is a deep hole in the sidewalk.
I fall in... I am helpless... It isn't my fault...
It takes forever to find a way out.

— act 2 —

I walk, down the street,
there is a deep hole in the sidewalk.
I pretend that I don't see it. I fall in again.
I can't believe I am in the same place,
but it isn't my fault.
It still take a long time to get out.

— act 3 —

I walk, down the street,
there is a deep hole in the sidewalk.
I see it is there. I still fall. It's a habit.
My eyes are open. I know where I am.
It is my fault. I get out immediately.

— act 4 —

I walk, down the street,
there is a deep hole in the sidewalk.
I walk around it.

— act 5 —

I walk down another street.

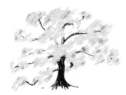

Monica Verplank
Chopra Center Certified Master Educator
Ayurvedic Life-Style Consultant
MonicaVerplank.com

Chapter 8.
Dealing with It: Your
Mind and Emotions

"Emancipate yourselves from mental slavery, none but ourselves can free our minds!"

— Bob Marley

As toxicity can accumulate in our physical life, it also can accumulate in our mental and emotional life. When we hold on to resentments and grievances, we continue to carry the psychoemotional burden by allowing a past incident to continue to affect us in the present. Numerous studies have shown that anger, loneliness, and isolation can have negative health consequences while gratitude and forgiveness can lead to health benefits. Controlling our mind and emotions can be a challenge, but it is possible to free yourself from the hold of toxic thoughts and emotions.

I am reminded of the Zen story of two traveling monks who meet a woman who is unable to cross a stream on her own. Without hesitation, the older monk picks her up on his back and carries her across, despite having taken a vow to not touch women. He gently places her down on the other side of the stream and they each go on their way. After several hours, the younger monk is still troubled by what had occurred and admonishes the older monk, "How could you do that? We are not supposed to make eye contact with women, let along pick them up and carry them!" To which the older monk replies, "Oh, are you still carrying her? I put her down when I reached the other side of the stream." How many upsets are you still carrying that no longer serve you?

If you are ready to let that stuff go, cultivating a meditative practice is a great place to start. While meditation and mindfulness have been found to have particular mental and physical benefits, people can achieve meditative states in a variety of ways. The key is to get to a place where you are free from clinging to the constant barrage of thoughts. Perhaps you might find that zone while running, painting, singing, or knitting; regularly tapping into this state of being can help pull us out of a reactive state where we are ruled by primitive emotions.

You may identify certain toxic thought patterns, emotions, or relationships that you recognize are no longer serving you. Freeing yourself from that emotional toxicity opens you up to healing. While I will give you some basic pointers here, I highly recommend working with a trained professional who can guide you through the process if needed. At times, this toxicity runs deep and may need to be addressed over a period of time.

Nurturing your mental and emotional environment provides a foundation for healthy relationships, mental flexibility, and a more peaceful and joyful life. For many, this is an area that needs daily attention—bringing in the "good" and letting go of the "bad" to detoxify our thoughts. This is not to say that bad stuff will not happen. Life is full of major and minor stresses, but it is our interpretation and our attachment to the memory of these events or our anxious projection into the future that can keep us stuck in a negative mindset. If you find yourself doing so, it is time to start practicing these tools to enjoy life in the present moment.

48. Practice Meditation or Mindfulness

Meditation is a practice that helps to calm the mind and allows us to be awake and aware, yet detached from our incessant thoughts. Many meditation techniques exist and recent studies have shown a multitude of health benefits with a regular meditation practice—from enhancing brain structure and function to up-regulating genes for healing and self-regulation while down-regulating genes involved in inappropriate inflammatory processes.

Studies have demonstrated that meditation helps to reduce feelings of anxiety and depression, improve attention and concentration, and benefit overall psychological well-being. Through imaging studies, long-term meditators have been found to have better preservation of brain regions associated with working memory and executive decision making. And research has shown that even after just eight weeks of a thirty-minute practice per day, structural changes occurred in the brains of novice meditators including areas associated with stress, memory, and empathy. Other studies have shown improvements in memory and mind-wandering after participation in a two-week training course and beneficial changes in mental health and gene expression associated with stress and immune responses after just five days of participation in a meditation retreat. Although the length of time of practice does seem to make a difference in effect size, it is encouraging that these changes can even be seen in people who have only been practicing for a short time. It is an exciting time in meditation research when modern scientific tools are being used to validate the many benefits of these ancient practices.

Beyond these great health benefits, a regular meditation practice allows you to be more responsive and less reactive. It gives you the space to calm down and get out of fight-or-flight mode where we may make a rash decision or react on the spot without consciously thinking about the consequences of our actions. In life-or-death situations these reactions can save us, but too often we go into these reactive responses when triggered by something that is not really dangerous, like when someone zips into the parking spot you have been patiently waiting for, or when your child drops an entire gallon of milk on the floor just as you are about to leave for work, or when you are late for an appointment and seem to be hitting every single red light possible. By regularly practicing being in a calm state of mind, it is easier to shift out of an instant reaction mode and instead pause and move forward with a conscious response. This is not to say that you won't ever get upset—we all experience joy and sorrow, pleasure and pain—but the way that you express your discomfort will begin to shift away from a fly-off-the-handle type of reaction. On occasion, you may have reactive moments, but as you witness the consequences and are aware of your role in the situation, you will recover more quickly than before.

When we are less reactive, we are able to make decisions and choices from a place of consciousness. This can open us up to consider whether the actions we are taking are life-enhancing and leading to more health and wellness or not. Are the choices that we're making protecting ourselves from or limiting exposure to toxins? And as we think about the food that we eat and the products that we purchase, consider their journey from where the ingredients or components started all the way to where they will end up at the end of their use, and notice if there are steps along the way that produce benefit or harm for us, for future generations, and for the planet. As we bring this awareness in, we might find areas where we can improve what we do around our homes, in our workplaces, at our children's schools, and throughout the community. When we recognize that we can make these conscious choices, we reclaim our sense of control over what ends up in our bodies and minds.

Breath Awareness Meditation

Sit in a quiet, comfortable place with your eyes closed or with a soft gaze. As you feel settled, begin to follow your breathing as it goes in and out. Allow yourself to breathe naturally, without trying to make it change or forcing a certain rhythm or speed. Just notice as you breathe in, and notice as you breathe out. If you observe that your attention has drifted to thoughts, sensations, or noises, just gently bring your focus back to your breath. Continue to follow your breath for the period of time you have set aside for meditation. Twenty to thirty minutes is recommended, however, sitting for ten minutes is better than not at all. After you are finished, sit and relax for a moment before resuming activity.

Simple Mindfulness Practice

Sit in a quiet, comfortable place with your eyes closed or with a soft gaze. Take three slow breaths in and out and then allow yourself to settle, breathing normally. Turn your attention to your sense of hearing and for a minute or so observe the sounds in your environment without judgment. What do you hear nearby? What is far away? Are the sounds loud or soft? What are their qualities? Next, shift your attention to your sense of touch. Notice how your body feels where you are sitting. Are you cool or warm? Notice the texture of your clothes. Is there a breeze or is the air still? Then shift your attention to your sense of smell. What aromas can you detect in your environment? Are the smells familiar? Do they remind you of anything? Finally, allow your eyes to open if they were closed previously and shift your attention to your sense of sight. What are some of the things that you see? Are you somewhere dark or light? What colors are you observing? Then, just sit and relax for a moment before resuming activity.

Take a Media Fast

For most of my life, the television was a constant fixture and was on any time that I was home. But when my daughter was an infant, I suddenly became more aware of the constant stream of violence and negativity that was barraging us and turned the

TV off, particularly the news. What I didn't recognize before was that while it may seem informing and even empowering, the media in all forms is designed to influence your behaviors, thoughts, and feelings—sometimes to the point of manipulation. Why was the news repeatedly reporting the same stories without any new information? Stress, anxiety, and worry are powerful feelings that can keep viewers glued to the screen. But is this helpful and necessary? And who has control over my emotional state? Are our ideas our own, or are they being presented to us by people we likely have never even met? From "fake news" to social media ads and posts, we should wonder who is behind the information we are consuming and what their endgame is.

For some, our digital lives may be even more consuming that our real lives, with people having real addictions to Facebook and the internet. How many times a day do you check your email? Facebook? Other media feeds? Even seemingly positive interactions can create stress. Many can feel burdened by the need to comment or "like" their friends' posts, which then becomes a time-sucking chore that takes away from family, school, work, and a social life. And there are many negative aspects of social media as well including cyberbullying, body image concerns, depression, and anxiety. How's your digital life going? Does it fill you with joy and pleasure? Or are you left feeling empty, alone, and pissed off?

In our house, at least once a year we have a "screen-free week" where we turn off all electronic media—TVs, computers, laptops, tablets, and smartphones—unless required for work or school. Even better is when we can go on vacation and disconnect completely. My kids always protest at first. But we end up spending more time talking with each other, playing outside or creating things indoors, and most of all, connecting face-to-face. If this seems too daunting to you, at least carve out some time during the day when you refrain from tuning in to electronic media. For instance, check your email three times a day instead of all day long. Don't leave the TV on in the background if you are not watching it or allow the next program to just run without you actively choosing it. Another strategy is to turn off all screens after a certain time—you just might even sleep better. Taking a media fast can be a great way to reconnect with what is meaningful in your life and develop a more conscious relationship with the media.

Tips to Incorporate Meditation and Mindfulness into Your Life:

- **Take a meditation course in-person or online. Learning from an experienced teacher is the best way to start your meditation practice. You can learn about mindfulness techniques, mantra meditation, and many other forms of meditation.**
- **Listen to a guided meditation. Many recordings are now available to help guide you through a meditation practice. See the Resources section for a few of my favorites.**
- **Meditate with a friend. Some find meditating with someone or meditating in a group to be beneficial.**
- **Use a meditation app. Some are guided meditations while others have meditation timers for you to do your own practice. Some apps have a social networking component that allow you to be part of a virtual meditation community.**
- **Meditate first thing in the morning. Getting it done as soon as you get up leaves no room for excuses.**
- **Use media with awareness. Consider taking a media fast.**

49. Forgiveness and Gratitude

Both forgiveness and gratitude have been linked to enhanced happiness and well-being. While practicing forgiveness can be a process that takes effort, daily gratitude practices can be relatively easy to accomplish.

The Freedom of Forgiveness

Throughout life, we experience disappointments and hurts both big and small. But when we are unable to forgive, we hold on to the negative feelings keeping us stuck. Not forgiving someone essentially keeps us locked in an emotional prison, tied to the person or event. You may think that by holding a grudge or resentment you are "making them pay," but in reality the person who is really being affected is you. From negative thoughts to physical illness, I have seen many patients whose emotional toxicity has been a significant obstacle in their path to wellness. Like Nelson Mandela once said, "Resentment is like drinking poison and then hoping it will kill your enemies." When you are finally able to forgive, releasing the attachment to the wounded feelings, it is like unlocking the prison door— and the person being set free is not the other person, but you.

Research on forgiveness has shown that learning to forgive reduces the amount of hurt, anger, stress, and depression that people experience. As you stop replaying the negative story, releasing bitterness, anger, resentment, and remorse, your brain is freed up to focus on more positive thoughts and relationships. People become more hopeful, optimistic, and compassionate and notice improved physical health as well. So with all of these benefits, why is it so hard?

Forgiveness is not about forgetting what happened. It isn't about justifying or condoning what the other person did or making someone else apologize or change. It is about your decision to let go of the impact of the event, setting yourself free from the emotional trigger so that you can move forward on your own terms. It is about finding peace and understanding. It is about changing the tone of your story, shifting from focusing on the hurt feelings that gives power to the other person who you perceived as causing your pain and instead opening up to the lessons, kindness, and love that can restore your personal power and strength. There are many ways to practice forgiveness and some people find working with a counselor or therapist to be helpful. When you are ready to let go of your emotional pain to set yourself free, I encourage you to embark on an emotional detox by practicing forgiveness.

The Gift of Gratitude

Like forgiveness, those who practice gratitude regularly experience an increase in joy, happiness, and overall satisfaction with their lives. In addition, research has shown potential health benefits: the ability to manage stress better; improved sleep, energy, and immune function; reduced inflammation; and improved heart health markers. A gratitude practice also can help mitigate isolation and loneliness which have been linked to increased health problems and higher mortality.

When we think about what we appreciate or are thankful for, we amplify positive memories and recruit other positive emotions that can favorably affect our physical and mental well-being. In addition, research has shown that when we think about what we are grateful for, we trigger the calming part of the nervous system (parasympathetic nervous system), which can also have positive health effects.

Take time to notice and reflect upon things that you are thankful for. You may want to keep a gratitude journal and write in it regularly. Choose a time that works for you to journal daily and commit to doing it. You don't need to drag out the practice for a long time, but aim to practice gratitude consistently. Try to notice new things that you are grateful for each day and get specific. Instead of just writing "I'm grateful for my family" over and over, think of something in particular about your family members such as, "My daughter stopped playing on her computer to give me a hug when she knew I was upset" or "My husband picked up dinner to give me a break." When we expand our awareness of the gifts in our life, we create a network of positive feelings and thoughts creating a ripple effect of health and well-being.

Tips to Practice Gratitude and Forgiveness:

- Practice gratitude daily by noticing what you are grateful for. Writing down what you are grateful for in a journal can be even more effective.
- If you recognize that you are holding on to emotional pain from a past event that is keeping you stuck, consider taking steps to free yourself of mental toxicity.

Chapter 9:
Beyond Ourselves:
Karma and
Consciousness

"The Earth is not just our environment. We are the Earth. The Earth is us."

- Thich Nhat Hahn

The world we live in now is the expression of our collective consciousness, and if we want a new world, we must each take responsibility in creating it. The first several chapters have focused on what you can to do minimize toxicity in your own personal environment. This is important because cleaning up areas in which you have control can greatly reduce your toxic exposures and toxic load. But we also have to go out into the community and into the world at large. And as you have learned, what is in the world spreads all over the world. Becoming conscious of the way that we live is a first step in environmental detoxification and personal responsibility. But don't just live in a protective cocoon, merely paying attention to yourself and your immediate environment—you must go beyond.

As you gain awareness of the extent of pollution affecting our entire planet, you may wonder what you can do to change the course of our current path of destruction. Practicing the three Rs of the environment—reduce, reuse, recycle—is a great place to start that makes an impact both on a personal and a global level. At a community level, consider what changes can be made in your neighborhood or in your children's schools. How can we inform our local and national government to make good choices that reduce pollution and promote health? What can be done to make regulations and industry standards in alignment with promoting health and preventing harm rather than lining the pockets of industries and corporations? And what can we do to shift the mindset of those industries? It takes effort to chip away little by little in all of these areas, but progress is being made by people like you continuing to educate themselves and spreading the word for change.

Once there are enough people sharing the same intention, a tipping point is reached and change occurs. We see evidence of the seeds of change in the organic and non-GMO food movements, in the increase in green technologies, and in curbside recycling and composting efforts. People are already paving the way for a collective shift for the good of all. Social media and the internet are breaking down barriers to information, creating virtual communities and alliances around the global community. As the collective consciousness shifts and spreads to others, momentum builds and can create big changes in the way things are done. I am inspired by the words of President Barack Obama: "Change will not come if we wait for some other person or some other time. We are the ones we've been waiting for. We are the change that we seek." It is time to be a part of that change.

50. Live the 3 Rs: Reduce, Reuse, Recycle

We are a nation of consumers, and all of the products that we purchase use resources to manufacture, transport, and sometimes even sell them—even those made from recycled materials. Then we treat most of what we purchase as disposable, throwing away fifty billion food and drink cans, twenty-seven billion glass bottles and jars, sixty-five million plastic and metal jar and can covers, thirteen million tons of textiles, and fifty billion plastic water bottles each year in America alone. And don't get me started on packaging materials, which make up more than a third of our waste and is often plastic, plus our use of 100 billion plastic and 10 billion paper shopping bags a year, using approximately 14 million trees and 12 million barrels of oil. The majority of this waste ends up in landfills where it can take hundreds or thousands of years to decompose or, in the case of plastics, never decompose at all. This is contributing to numerous environmental problems in landfills, incinerators, the phenomenon of the Great Pacific Garbage Patch, and microplastics in water around the world. The problem with waste is that even though we don't necessarily see it, it doesn't actually go away. Therefore, we need to do our part to practice three Rs of the environment: reduce, reuse, and recycle. Doing so can save energy, natural resources, and money while also protecting the environment.

"Reduce" means using fewer resources and is the most effective of the three Rs. One step is to cut back on your consumption. Simply put, don't buy things that you don't need. See if you can borrow, rent, or share rather than purchase an item you might use infrequently. Resist the temptation to buy all the latest fads which quickly go out of fashion. Instead of "disposable" products, look for things that will last. The money that you spend on well-made, durable products will offset the cost of replacing cheap, throwaway items. Keeping things maintained and repaired also means they won't have to be thrown out or replaced as often. Steer away from wasteful packaging and buy in bulk when you can. Stop junk mail by asking to be removed from the distribution list.

Another aspect of "reduce" is purchasing products that use fewer resources such as choosing energy-efficient appliances, electronics, and vehicles; purchasing products made from recycled materials such as paper and bathroom tissue; and buying locally sourced or produced items that use less energy for transportation. Avoid items which are made with materials that are obtained by destructive extraction or processing techniques such as tropical woods and most gold jewelry. We can reduce our use of resources in the home as well by cutting back on water use, monitoring our use of energy and shutting off electronics and lights when not in use, and reducing the amount of waste going to landfills by composting and recycling. Reduce the use of cars by carpooling, walking, biking, or taking public transportation when you can. Consider installing solar panels to reduce dependence on fossil fuels for energy and possibly lower energy costs.

To reduce energy usage, OhmConnect is a new service that monitors real-time conditions on the electricity grid. When dirty and unsustainable power plants turn on, users receive a notification to conserve energy. If additional power plants do not have to be turned on, we reduce resources and costs, and OhmConnect has gamified energy saving by providing ways to earn points and money through their app.

"Reuse" means considering whether an item can still be used in some way before being recycled or put into the waste stream. While many items can be reused as is (books, magazines, DVDs, clothes, and furniture), the creative part is discovering new uses that may be different from the original use—food scraps can become compost, an old towel can become a rag, an opened envelope can become a shopping list, a food jar can be used for storage, a plastic water bottle can be cut into plastic rope. Reusing keeps these items from entering the waste stream and holds off on using resources for new items. Gently used items can also be donated or consigned, and many organizations such as local churches, community centers, thrift stores, schools, and nonprofit organizations accept donated items. As an added bonus, you may receive a tax benefit by donating items. If you are looking to purchase items, you can find used clothes, household items, electronics, building materials, and cars—often at a much lower price than if bought new. Items can also be made into new products through upcycling or repurposing.

"Recycling" is the process of collecting and processing materials that would otherwise be thrown away as trash and turning them into new products. Look for products made from recycled materials when purchasing new items to keep the cycle going. Because of curbside recycling programs that make this easier, this "R" has caught on the best, but there is still a lot that can be done to make it better. Each municipality has its own rules about what can or cannot be recycled, so pay attention to what types of plastics and other materials are accepted. Just seeing the recycling chasing arrow symbol on the bottom of a container does not mean that it is appropriate to put it into the recycling bin. In fact, the wrong kind of plastic can contaminate a whole batch due to being incompatible with a different melting point, making the entire batch garbage to the recycling company and negating all of your good efforts. For instance, while a clean pizza box can be recycled and often has a recycling symbol on it, pizza boxes and any paper product that is stained with grease or food are not recyclable. During the recycling process, grease from pizza boxes causes oil to form at the top of a slurry, and paper fibers cannot separate from oils, which ruins the batch. My family may think I'm an obsessive-compulsive recycler, diving after greasy pizza boxes in the recycling bin and clean pasta boxes in the trash, but there is a reason why these recycling rules exist, and it is important to learn the recycling rules in your own community.

Here's the lowdown on some of the top recycled items:

Paper. Makes up nearly 30 percent of waste, more than any other material. Check what is accepted before putting paper and paper products into the recycling bin—for instance, many paper cups are lined with plastic that keeps them from becoming soggy, but makes them non-recyclable. Look for products made from recycled paper when purchasing.

Plastics. These make up about 13 percent of waste and some types of plastics are recycled more than others. Most community recycling programs accept some types of plastics, but not all. So it is important to look at the numbers on the bottom of the container and follow the rules of your recycling program.

Glass. Most community recycling programs accept different glass colors and types mixed together, but check to see if you need to sort your glass.

Batteries. Because they often contain heavy metals such as mercury, lead, cadmium, and nickel, batteries should not be thrown out in the regular trash. Lead-acid car batteries can be returned to stores that sell car batteries and then may be recycled. Check your waste management program to find the best way to dispose of other batteries used in electronics.

Motor Oil. The used oil from one oil change can contaminate one million gallons of fresh water, so never dump used motor oil down the drain. It takes one gallon of used oil versus forty-two gallons of crude oil to produce 2.5 quarts of new motor oil, so recycling can make a big impact. Check with auto-supply stores and repair shops to see if they will accept motor oil for recycling.

Household Hazardous Waste (HHW) and Electronics. Products that contain corrosive, toxic, ignitable, or reactive ingredients are considered to be HHW. Paints, cleaners, oils, batteries, CFL bulbs, computers, and pesticides require special care when you dispose of them as they may be dangerous to people or the environment. These should not be thrown out with regular trash, poured down the drain, or dumped on the ground. Check with your waste management agency to see how to dispose of HHW. Communities often have special collection and recycling events for these types of products.

Tips to Follow the 3 Rs:

- **Invest in well-made, durable products, and keep them maintained and repaired.**
- **Buy in bulk and steer away from wasteful packaging.**
- **Bring your reusable bags when you go shopping. Use reusable containers to bring lunch and for food storage.**
- **Remove yourself from junk mail distribution lists by writing to the Direct Marketing Association.**
- **Purchase products that use fewer resources such as those that are recycled, upcycled, reused, energy-efficient, or locally made.**
- **Reduce personal use of resources by cutting back on purchasing new items, reducing waste, cutting back on water use, and being more energy-efficient.**
- **Donate, consign, or reuse items which still have life left in them.**
- **Take advantage of curbside recycling programs and check with waste management to see how to properly dispose of or recycle items. Learn what CAN be recycled and don't put items in recycling bins that do not belong there.**

51. Support Companies Doing Good

It can be overwhelming to think of going up against the big polluters in our society—the big industry giants with deep pockets and political influence—who want to keep doing what they are doing without taking responsibility for the consequences. Focused on the short-term goal of selling us a product, many companies either are not aware or do not care that some aspect of their business may actually be causing harm to the environment and to human health. But a growing number of companies see the rising consumer demand for sustainability and environmental responsibility and are answering the call.

Today's consumers want to know where their products are coming from, what they are made of, and who is making them. They are looking for safer, natural products and are often willing to pay more for them, especially parents of young children. This demand has caused a growth since 2012 of 35 percent in US sales of beauty, household, and personal care products that make natural claims versus 4 percent for the broader industry. On the surface, this looks like good news, but unfortunately no regulatory guidelines currently exist for what makes a household product "natural," and labels can be deceptive as manufacturers are not required to disclose their ingredients for certain products. This has spawned an industry of "greenwashing"—claiming a product is eco-friendly, non-toxic, hypoallergenic, vegetable-based, natural, etc.—when it may contain many of the same harmful ingredients that are the same as mainstream products. The term "organic" is more stringent and ingredients must be certified by an independent body that follows USDA guidelines, but I have seen many products using certified organic ingredients mixed in alongside toxic ingredients.

So it is up to you the consumer to read the labels, ask questions, and vote with your wallet. As consumer demand shifts, so do the offerings at retailers. For instance, in 2015 Costco surpassed Whole Foods as the largest organic retailer. Companies like Kroger and Walmart have expanded their organic offerings; Target is working on more sustainable products including reducing waste from packaging. But these convenient big-box stores still contribute to a lot of waste and toxicity, and while they may offer big bargains, you may consider the question, "What is the real cost of purchasing this item?" When you consider the whole life cycle of a product—from how it is manufactured, to how it is used and disposed of—then you can make an informed choice. With these decisions, each individual can play a role in a new economic revolution that values health, wellness, and sustainability over toxic, cheap products that bring temporary happiness or convenience.

Tips to Support Companies Doing Good:
- **Read labels and beware of "greenwashed" products.**
- **Look at the company behind the product and support those with values in line with your own.**
- **Support local and smaller, independently-owned companies that promise accountability.**

52. The Karma of Consciousness

When we hear about climate change and global warming, it can be easy to tune out and think, "What can I possibly do about this?" or "That's too bad about the Earth, but back to me and my life … ." What I think is missing in this conversation is the recognition that the Earth and us are not separate—we are interconnected and interdependent. And so, as we are becoming conscious to the health status of our planet, we are waking up to an alarming and inconvenient truth. The chemicals of the last century, designed to make our lives easier, more convenient, cleaner, and brighter, are poisoning our planet and poisoning ourselves. No one on this planet is able to escape this toxicity.

One way to think about this issue is in terms of karma, which is a word that is sometimes misunderstood, but in simplified terms just means action. When we see karma in play, we can observe that what we have done in the past determines the consequences of how things are now arising. The world we live in now is a result of past actions. But we have an opportunity to break free from predictable, conditioned responses and determine our future by becoming aware. When we are more aware, the choices that we make in the present moment and the intentions that we have for the future are not determined by our past but emerge from our creative source. Conscious choice-making is the most effective way of creating future beneficial consequences of karma. It is summarized simply by the proverb, "As we sow, so shall we reap." If we continue to pollute the planet with garbage and toxic chemicals, we will see the effects of the garbage and chemicals in us as disease. On the other hand, if we plant seeds of health, harmony, and well-being with our actions and intentions, caring for and purifying our environment on all levels, then we will see the results of a clean and healthy life. For example, since DDT was banned because of the harm it was causing to humans and wildlife, we have seen a resurgence of bald eagles that had been decimated by this toxic substance and are now able to recover. The key to karma is understanding that you are responsible for your actions and that your actions can have both long-term and short-term consequences.

We are creating the world we live in through the choices we make every single day. Start to ask yourself questions: Who made this? What is it made of? Where did it come from, and where will it go when I'm done with it? How do I know it is safe? Do I really need it? Is there a safer or more eco-friendly way to do this? Toxicity should not have to be a consumer choice. Let your voice be heard by shopping according to your values. Let your neighbors and public officials know that these issues are important to you. We need to regain some control over what ends up in our bodies and say "no" to systems that allow people and the planet to be poisoned. The major health issues that we face today are connected to our lifestyle in a web of consequences from our dependence on fossil fuels to toxic products made from oil by-products, from soil-depleting conventional farming practices to cheap, nutrient-poor foods, from our yearning for cheap, endless resources to the pollution of our finite and necessary natural resources of air, earth, and water.

Say "yes" to preserving and protecting our natural resources, to supporting sustainable use, and to promoting an economy that values life, health, and well-being. When we all do our part, acting with awareness and intention, we begin to move the needle back to balance. As Margaret Mead said, "Never doubt that a small group of thoughtful, committed citizens can change the world."

Karma in Action:

- **Consider the decisions that you make in your daily life and lean towards choices that are life-enhancing for you and for the planet.**
- **Think about the downstream consequences of your actions.**
- **Share these ideas with friends and family.**
- **Align your purchases with your values. Consider what you are ultimately supporting with your money.**
- **Let your government know what you feel is important by voting, attending town halls, and writing or calling your representing officials locally and nationally.**

Putting It All Together: The Resilient Plan

By following the Action Steps that I have presented in this plan, you will reduce toxic exposures from your food, personal care products, clothing, home and garden, and community. You will also optimize your ability to handle toxins by following my Toxin Tamer Tips to improve your physical as well as mental digestion, detoxification, and elimination. Having helped thousands of clients on their path to health and healing, I know the importance of addressing each and every layer in order to get the best results. But even if you only incorporate some of the suggestions, you will be improving your state of health.

As you progress on your journey, it is my hope that you will start to incorporate the concepts of awareness, assessment, and action which provided the main sections of the book and which were also incorporated into each Action Step. For each choice that you make, becoming aware of the options, assessing what lies behind it and what the potential outcomes may be, and then acting based on this information will allow you to make conscious decisions. And if you make conscious choices, chances are they will also be evolutionary choices that will move you and the planet towards greater well-being.

Appendix A: Basic Elimination Diet Guide

An elimination diet is a great tool to determine if certain foods are creating negative reactions in your body that can lead you to feel poorly or even contribute to illness. While true food allergies that cause IgE responses leading to rashes, digestive issues, and possibly anaphylaxis can be tested for with a blood or skin test, other types of food sensitivities may be more difficult to identify. Some of the symptoms of eating foods to which you are sensitive include digestive disturbances (gas, bloating, heartburn), irritable bowel symptoms (constipation, loose stools, diarrhea), fatigue, inability to lose weight, joint pain, skin disorders, hormonal imbalances, and brain fog. By identifying and eliminating these trigger foods, people can experience a reduction of symptoms and overall better health. After identifying and eliminating their food sensitivities my patients have noticed increased energy, better digestion, improved hormonal balance, clearer skin, more restful sleep, better focus and concentration, reduced pain, and weight loss.

Complete the Food Sensitivity Questionnaire before you start the Elimination Diet and after completion of the Elimination Diet.

Food Sensitivity Questionnaire

Do you experience on a regular basis (i.e., more than 3 times a week):	Before	After
Abdominal bloating/distension		
Frequent burping or belching		
Abdominal cramps		
Abdominal or stomach pain		
Feeling nauseated after eating		
Feeling sluggish or tired after eating		
Excessive gas (flatulence)		
Indigestion		
Heartburn or Gastro-Esophageal Reflux Disease (GERD)		
Irregular bowel movements (constipation or diarrhea)		
Irritable Bowel Syndrome (IBS)		
Anal itching		
Hemorrhoids		
Sinus congestion or runny nose		
Ear congestion		
Throat itching, sore throat, or frequent need to clear throat		
Rash or other sores		
Acne		
Water retention		
Brain fog		
Inability to concentrate or focus		
Food cravings		
Fatigue		
Moodiness		
Sleep disturbance/insomnia		
Joint pain		
Fibromyalgia		

Headaches		
Inability to lose weight despite physical activity and "healthy" diet		
What is your weight?		
What is your waist circumference?		
What is your hip circumference?		

If you answered yes to one or more of the questions, then trying an elimination diet may be helpful for you to identify potential food triggers for your symptoms. The most common foods to which people are sensitive include:

- Gluten (wheat and other gluten grains)
- Dairy
- Soy
- Eggs
- Corn
- Peanuts
- Artificial sweeteners/flavorings/colors

By eliminating these foods from your diet for 21 days, you will cleanse your body of any "reactivities" that may have been caused by these substances. If you know or suspect that you have other food sensitivities or allergies (such as to nuts), then those foods should also be removed. Some of the other foods my patients have found they were sensitive to include citrus, yeast, nightshade vegetables, high-lectin foods, or caffeine. In addition, heavy consumption of sugar can wreak havoc on multiple systems in the body and increase inflammation, so reducing sugar consumption during this time is also important. And since you are making the effort to clean things up, choosing organic items (particularly for foods on the EWG Dirty Dozen list) and less toxic animal products is also advised.

For full benefit, it is important to be 100 percent compliant with the diet for the full three weeks. This allows the body's detoxification and elimination processes, which may be overburdened or compromised, to recover and begin to function efficiently again. Even consuming a small amount of a substance to which you are sensitive can create a whole cascade of reactions in your body leading to dysfunction. By adhering to this diet for the full twenty-one days, you will likely experience a notable shift in how you feel as you will have reduced inflammation and cleared immune complexes throughout your body.

The first three days of the elimination diet tend to be the most difficult. Since this may be a new way of eating for you, be sure to prepare in advance by going to the grocery store and planning out your menus for the first three to seven days, including snacks. Refer to the suggested foods, recipes, and food substitution resources. You may experience some physical discomfort initially related to detoxification which could include headache, bowel changes, joint or muscle aches, changes in sleep patterns, fatigue, and lightheadedness. These symptoms rarely last for more than a few days and if so should be evaluated by a healthcare practitioner. It is important to maintain excellent hydration with pure water and to have regular bowel movements daily. After seven days, you will have gotten used to the diet and should start to see improvements in how you feel.

After completely eliminating these foods for twenty-one days, you'll reassess how you feel using the Food Sensitivity Questionnaire again and then compare it to your baseline results. The next phase is to re-challenge your body by carefully reintroducing the foods in a systematic way to see if they provoke any symptoms. If they do cause any symptoms, then it will be important to remove these items from your diet for a longer period of time. If they do not cause symptoms, then they can be fully reintroduced back into your diet.

If you have no improvement at all after three weeks and do not have any symptom exacerbation upon re-challenge, either you do not have any sensitivities to these particular foods, or you may still have sensitivities but another factor is complicating your picture.

What to Eat During the Elimination Diet:

- Include fresh fruits and vegetables, non-gluten grains, tree nuts/seeds/oils, beans/legumes, and lean sources of protein.
- Try to eat at least three servings of fresh vegetables each day. Choose at least one serving of dark green or orange vegetables (carrots, broccoli, winter squash). Vary your selections.
- Eat organic fruits and vegetables if possible. See the EWG list of those most likely to have high amounts of pesticides: www.ewg.org/foodnews/list/
- If you select animal sources of protein, look for free-range or organically raised. If choosing fish, select wild-caught.
- For vegetarian option, eliminate the meats and fish and consume more beans, rice, and non-gluten grains (amaranth, millet, quinoa, sorghum, teff, buckwheat, gluten-free oats)
- Drink the recommended amount of plain, filtered water each day. At least two quarts of water or half your ideal body weight in ounces.
- Avoid any foods that you know or believe you may be sensitive to, even if they are on the "allowed" list.
- Avoid items listed below with a * if you may have a reaction to them. Otherwise, if doing a basic elimination, these foods are allowed.

	INCLUDE THESE FOODS	AVOID THESE FOODS
FRUIT	Whole fruits (berries), unsweetened frozen or water-packed fruits, unsweetened dried fruits (limit amount), unsweetened juices (limit amount)	Minimize high glycemic fruits: banana, grapes, mango, papaya, pineapple, watermelon *Oranges, *orange juice *other citrus
VEGETABLES	All vegetables: raw, juiced, steamed, sautéed, stir-fried, or roasted	Corn, creamed vegetables, or vegetables with cheese sauce *Nightshade vegetables: tomatoes, potatoes, eggplants, peppers (black or white pepper as a spice is okay), paprika, salsa, chili peppers, cayenne, chili powder
LEGUMES, BEANS	Lentils, split peas, legumes, beans	Soybeans and soybean products, soy sauce, soybean oil, tempeh, tofu, soy milk, soy yogurt, textured vegetable protein

| NUTS & SEEDS | Coconut, pine nuts, flax seeds, avocado | Peanuts, peanut butter

*Sesame, pump-kin, and sunflower seeds; tree nuts (walnuts, hazel-nuts, pecans, almonds, cashews); and nut butters (including tahini) |
|---|---|---|
| OILS | Cold-pressed extra-virgin olive oil, coco-nut oil, flaxseed oil, canola oil, grapeseed oil, organic ghee | Butter, margarine, shortening, pro-cessed oils, corn oils, vegetable oils, soybean oil

*Sesame, safflower, sunflower, and walnut oils |
| ANIMAL PROTEIN | Lamb, wild game, duck, organic chicken and turkey; wild-caught fresh, frozen, or water-packed canned fish | Canned meats, luncheon meats/cold cuts, sausage, frankfurters, hot dogs

*Pork, beef/veal, shellfish |
| OTHER PROTEIN | Rice, pea, hemp protein | Whey protein, soy protein

*Potato protein |

DAIRY & EGGS	Dairy substitutes such as rice milk, hemp milk, coconut milk	All dairy products: milk, cheese, yogurt, cream, non-dairy creamers; eggs and egg products *Almond milk, almond cheese
CONDIMENTS	Salt, pepper, and other spices, vinegar (balsamic, white/red wine, ume plum, apple cider), soy-free Veganaise, organic ketchup (check ingredients), coconut aminos	Mayonnaise, ketchup, store-bought relish, soy sauce, teriyaki sauce, store-bought BBQ sauce
SWEETENERS	Use only sparingly: fruit, maple syrup, blackstrap molasses, green leaf stevia (check ingredients and avoid if there are other added sweeteners), honey	Refined sugar, white/brown sugars, corn syrup, high-fructose corn syrup, evaporated cane juice
GRAINS AND STARCH	Rice, millet, quinoa, amaranth, teff, tapioca, buckwheat, gluten-free oats, arrowroot flour	Wheat, barley spelt, rye, triticale, faro, corn *Potato flour

Preparation for the Twenty-One Days

Prepare by reviewing all of the materials beforehand and going shopping to get all of the foods that you are allowed to have.

Make sure to read all labels carefully to find hidden culprits (see Hidden Sources section). Eat a wide variety of foods and do not try to restrict your calorie intake. Eat foods under the "Include These Foods" and avoid those under "Avoid These Foods" lists. If you are used to regularly consuming caffeine and decide to eliminate it as well, decrease your consumption gradually to avoid symptoms of withdrawal. Taking 1,000 mg of buffered vitamin C with breakfast and dinner may help reduce symptoms of caffeine withdrawal. Adequate rest and stress reduction is also important to the success of this program. Strenuous or prolonged exercise may be reduced during some of or the entire program to allow the body to heal more effectively without the additional burden imposed by exercise.

Reduce or eliminate any non-prescribed vitamin, mineral, or herbal supplements, particularly those that contain dairy, gluten, soy, or corn products. If you are taking many daily supplements, reduce use gradually over a seven-to-ten-day period before starting the Elimination Diet. For many of my patients, I recommend supplements by Pure Encapsulations, which are free of these ingredients. To order online, go to: www.valenciaporter.com/supplements/

Before you begin the program, prepare your family and friends by explaining what you plan to do and asking for their support. If everyone in your household agrees to eat the foods recommended on this diet when eating at home, it will be easier for you to stick to it by providing support as well as simplifying meal preparation. Review the list of foods (and hidden sources) that will be eliminated from your diet and put them away, give them away, or throw them away. Give perishables away or move them to the back of the bottom shelf in your refrigerator if they will not spoil. Move other non-perishables out of sight.

The First Three Days

The first two to three days can be difficult for some people. Different reactions may occur, especially in the first week as the body adjusts to a different dietary regimen. Anytime you change your diet significantly, you may experience symptoms such as fatigue, headache, light-headedness, muscle aches, sleep changes, or constipation for a few days. In addition you may crave some foods that you are used to consuming. Be patient, as these symptoms usually resolve after the first several days. If they don't resolve, then you should seek a healthcare practitioner for further evaluation.

Make sure your bowels are moving regularly. If you are having difficulty, try drinking warm water with lemon juice first thing in the morning. Magnesium citrate 300 to 600 mg or Triphala 1000 mg to 2000 mg at night may be helpful for constipation when indicated.

Tips for Success

- Plan your meals ahead. Eat simply. Cook simply.
- Reduce packaged, processed, and prepared foods, which are more likely to have hidden culprits. Make foods yourself, so that you know exactly what is in it. Read the ingredients for anything that comes in a package or that you have not made yourself from scratch, including canned and frozen foods.
- Have food on hand so you can grab something quickly without having to think about it. Keep your blood sugar stable by eating meals regularly, and if necessary have a healthy snack between meals. Carry allowed foods with you when you leave the house. That way you will have what you are allowed and not be tempted to stray off the plan.
- Make foods easily available and ready-to-eat or ready-to-prepare. Prepare extra rice or quinoa to easily add to a stir-fry, a bowl, or other meals. Cook extra chicken, sweet potatoes, beans, etc., that can be reheated for snacking or another meal. Make a pot of chicken-vegetable-rice soup. Fix a large salad.

- Change your concept of breakfast. Typical breakfast foods abound with wheat, eggs, and dairy and often look more like a dessert. You might have to think outside of the box of what breakfast typically looks like—many other parts of the world typically have more of a savory, protein-rich breakfast. Try to ensure that you get some protein. Smoothies with berries and non-dairy, non-soy protein (hemp, pea, or rice protein) are often the easiest solution.

- Try to start the diet at a time where you are free from social engagements and when stress levels are low in order to make the adjustment easier. If for some reason you must break the diet, treat the occasion as a food challenge, and then resume the elimination diet. Record food consumption and any symptoms that occur

- Be careful when eating out—particularly with sauces and condiments—and ask how things are prepared. For example butter, containing dairy, can sometimes be added to steaks after grilling to enhance their flavor, or something appearing gluten-free may be cooked on the same grill as something prepared in wheat flour, thus leaving small amounts of gluten residue on your food. Safe options include plain steamed or sautéed vegetables and plain grilled fish, poultry, or meat (you can ask about oil and seasoning options for both) or a salad with oil and vinegar as a dressing. Having a pre-written list of the foods you cannot have may be helpful:

Dear Chef,

For health reasons, I cannot eat:

- Wheat/gluten
- Dairy
- Soy
- Eggs
- Corn
- Peanuts
- Artificial sweeteners/flavorings/colors
- _____
- _____
- _____
- _____

Thank you for your assistance in helping me avoid these items in my meal.

Carry a list with you of food items that you will not be eating to inform anyone else who will be preparing your foods.

Food Challenge: Bringing the Eliminated Foods Back

Once you have eliminated a food or food group from your diet for at least three weeks, then reintroducing the food as a challenge item will allow you to see if you are sensitive to that food. Often these are the foods that you crave the most. You may have already noticed an improvement in your symptoms during the elimination phase of the diet. Reintroducing a food to which you are intolerant or sensitive may retrigger those symptoms. If you identify specific food intolerances, you will then need to continue to keep the food item out of your diet for a minimum of six months. It is also important to seek the advice of a health care practitioner who is knowledgeable about handling food intolerances and sensitivities to help with gut recovery and address other potential imbalances and symptoms which may have resulted from eating these foods in the past.

If you have had no improvement after three weeks, then there are a few possibilities to explain this: 1) Some people notice little change on the elimination phase but then do notice a distinct worsening when re-challenging with an offending food. Therefore, completing the challenge part of this diet is still worthwhile. 2) You may not have any sensitivities to the foods which were eliminated. This elimination diet focuses on the most likely culprits, but others include citrus, yeast, nightshade vegetables, high-lectin foods, and caffeine. If you do the food re-challenge and still have not identified any sensitivities, you may choose to do a new elimination diet with any of these additional food groups or consider detailed food sensitivity testing with a health care practitioner. 3) You may still have sensitivities, but other contributing factors prevented an improvement in your symptoms with only diet change. Potential factors which may contribute to a more complex problem include impairments in your detoxification system, hormonal imbalance, immune dysfunction, microbial imbalance, or underlying disease. To address these, it is important to seek the advice of a health care practitioner who can evaluate any underlying causes.

How to Do a Food Challenge

In this next phase, you will carefully add foods back into your diet one at a time to see which foods may be triggering symptoms. This part of the program is called the Challenge Phase because you are challenging your body to handle foods that most often cause symptoms. Again, if you have no bad reaction when reintroducing the food, your body has met the challenge and proven that it can handle that food. But if you do have an adverse reaction, then you have identified one of your problem foods that you should then avoid.

Add back only one food at a time, starting with the foods that are least likely to be causing symptoms. Do not add back foods which have combinations of items until they have all been cleared. For example, bread would not be a good challenge item until eggs, dairy, and wheat have been cleared. Continue to read your labels. Below is a suggested order to reintroduce foods, but if you suspect that you have a sensitivity to a particular food, then try that food last.

1. Corn
2. Eggs
3. Gluten (Wheat)
4. Dairy
5. Peanuts
6. Soy
(I don't recommend adding back the artificial stuff)

What to Do

Eat the challenge food at least twice a day and in a fairly large amount for at least two to three days. Try to eat the food at each meal. For example, for corn you could eat Simply Maize Organic Corn Cereal for breakfast, tacos with corn tortillas for lunch, corn chips for a snack, and salad with fresh corn at dinner. An offending food may provoke symptoms within ten minutes to twelve hours, sometimes longer. Look for symptoms such as headache, bloating, nausea, diarrhea, indigestion, fatigue, feeling tired after a meal, flushing, rapid heartbeat, dizziness, and itching. If you do not notice any reaction, continue to challenge with this food for two to three days total. Use the Food Sensitivity Questionnaire to compare symptoms to your baseline.

If you do have a reaction to the food, then remove that food from your diet for at least two days to more than a week before introducing a new challenge food. Wait until your symptoms have completely subsided before challenging with the next food.

You will then want to keep that food out of your diet for at least six months and perhaps even longer. For example, you may introduce corn with no problem, but then you introduce eggs and have a reaction. You would stop eating eggs and continue with the allowed elimination diet foods, now including corn, which you had found you were able to tolerate. Stay on this program until you have no further reactions and your body has recovered, then you will reintroduce the next food on the list, keeping eggs and egg products out of your diet for the next six months. It is advisable that you seek the advice of a health care practitioner who is versed in managing food sensitivities and healing gut function to determine your next steps if you do have a food reaction. By avoiding symptom-provoking foods and taking supportive supplements to restore gut integrity, microbial balance, and immune function, it is possible that food sensitivities may resolve or diminish after some time. If that occurs, you would then be able to eat some foods that formerly caused problems. In some cases, however, the sensitivity may take longer to resolve or may remain long-term.

If you do not have a reaction after two to three days of consistently eating the food, then you likely do not have a sensitivity to that food. Rarely, people have a delayed reaction up to a week after bringing the food back into the diet. If you don't react you may then continue to eat that food in regular portions. Try to keep these foods in rotation and don't consume them at high levels on a regular basis. You now have been familiarized with other alternatives that you can weave into your regular diet to avoid becoming sensitive to these foods in the future. I also recommend choosing the non-GMO, organic, and less processed versions of these foods

Tips for Success with the Food Challenge:
- Continue eating the foods that were allowed during the twenty-one-day Elimination Phase.
- Introduce only one food group at a time.

- Keep a daily journal of all foods eaten and all symptoms, including weight. Download a copy the Food Sensitivity Questionnaire at www.valenciaporter.com/foodsensitivity to track possible symptoms.
- Be sure to test foods in a pure form: for example, test milk or cheese or wheat, but not pizza, which contains milk, cheese, and wheat; eat cream-of-wheat instead of bread, which contains wheat, eggs, and milk.
- Continue to read food labels. Continue to avoid processed and packaged foods because they usually contain a combination of many ingredients. Do not reintroduce any food that contains a problem ingredient that has not yet been reintroduced.
- If you are unsure, take the food back out of your diet for at least one week and then re-challenge again. You may increase the amount of the food that you eat during the challenge.

CAUTION: Never do elimination/challenge testing on a food to which you have known or suspected life-threatening (anaphylactic) reactions. Persons with potentially life threatening conditions such as severe depression, severe asthma, seizures, extremely high blood pressure, heart arrhythmias, or other symptoms of a severe nature are not candidates for this at-home method of testing without medical supervision. The symptoms provoked on this diet may be more severe and dramatic than those experienced on an everyday chronic basis.

Hidden Sources of Foods

See the following tables for items that may contain these foods and keywords to look for to avoid these foods.

Gluten is a type of protein found in wheat (wheatberries, durum, emmer, semolina, spelt, farina, farro, graham,

kamut, and einkorn), rye, barley and triticale. Unless clearly labeled gluten-free, assume these items contain gluten:

• Alcohol made with grain, beer, ale, lager	• Chutneys	• Malt (including malt extract, flavoring, syrup, vinegar, and drinks)
• Baked beans	• Corn bread, corn muffins	
• Baked goods (cakes, cookies, muffins, pastry or pie crust, scones)	• Couscous	• Matzoh meal/ flour
	• Crackers, crispbreads	• Meat paste
• Biscuits	• Crumble toppings	• Meat dishes (prepackaged)
• Blue cheeses (may be made with bread)	• Doughnuts	• Muesli
	• Dumplings	• Mustard - dry mustard powder may contain
• Bread and bread rolls (wheat, white, whole grain, oat, rye bread, pumpernickel), breadcrumbs, breaded anything (such as meats)	• Falafel	
	• Fish paste	
	• Gravy powders and stock cubes such as bouillon	• Oats, oat bran, oat syrup (due to processing)
	• Hot dogs	• Orzo
• Brewer's yeast	• Hydrolyzed vegetable protein (HVP)	• Ovaltine
• Brown rice syrup (from barley caramel coloring)	• Imitation crab meat, imitation meat, imitation seafood	• Packaged mixes
		• Pancakes, waffles
• Bulgar/Bulgur	• Instant coffee (may be bulked out with flour)	• Pasta, noodles
• Candy		• Pates
• Cereals, cereal binding	• Licorice	• Pickles (in malt vinegar)
• Chapati flour (atta)	• Luncheon meat	• Pizza
• Chocolate, cocoa drinks		• Popovers
		• Postum

(Continued)

• Potato crisps/ chips (may have flour added) • Pretzels • Salad dressings • Sauces (flour as thickener) • Sausages • Seitan ("wheat meat") • Self-basting turkeys • Souffles • Soups (flour as thickener)	• Soy sauce • Spices: curry powder, white pepper, and other dried herbs and spices (can have added flour) • Stuffings • Suet (shredded in packs) • Textured vegetable protein (TVP)	• Vanilla extract (may contain) • Veggie chips • Vinegar (may be from wheat, malt) • Wheat (including bran, germ, starch) • White flour • Yorkshire pudding

Corn Ingredients in Foods

Other forms of corn used in foods	Hidden sources of corn
• Corn alcohol • Corn flour, corn meal • Corn oil, Mazola • Cornstarch (mazena) • Corn sugar, corn sweetener, corn syrup, corn syrup solids • Dextrose, dextrin • Grits • High fructose corn syrup, fructose, fructose syrup • Hominy	• Bacon (may have added corn product) • Baking powder • Beverages (corn syrup) • Candy • Corn containing cereals, corn flakes • Corn Batters, corn breads, corn muffins • Corn Chips • Ketchup • Mayonnaise (may have vinegar from corn)

• Maize, masa	• Peanut Butter (may contain corn syrup)
• Maltodextrins	
• Modified gum starch, modified food starch	• Processed foods (corn syrup, high fructose corn syrup, fructose syrup)
• Popcorn	
• Powdered sugar	• Tortillas and tortilla chips (made from corn)
• Sorbitol	
• Starch (food, vegetable, modified food starch)	• Vegetable oil
	• Envelope and stamp adhesive
• Vegetable gum	
• Vinegar (may be from corn)	• Toothpaste

Dairy foods include cow, goat and sheep milks, yogurts and cheeses

Dairy may be listed as:	Hidden sources of dairy	
• Milk	• Artificial butter flavor	• Gravies
• Milk solids		• Hard sauces
• Milk proteins	• Au gratin or "scalloped" dishes	• Hot dogs
• Non-fat milk solids	• Bavarian cream	• Ice Cream, sherbet
	• Many baked goods: biscuits, breads, crackers, cakes, cookies, doughnuts	• Kefir
• Casein		• Malted milk
• Caseinate		• Mashed potatoes (prepared with milk and/or butter)
• Lactose		
• Lactalbumin		
• Sodium caseinate	• Many baking mixes (pancake mix)	• Meat and deli meats (casein may be used as a binder)
• Whey		• Meat loaf
	• Butter and many margarines	• Many "non-dairy" products (coffee creamer, whipped topping)

(Continued)

• Buttermilk or buttermilk solids	•
• Candy	• Omelets
• Canned foods (soups, spaghetti, ravioli)	• Ovaltine
• Cheese, cream cheese, cottage cheese	• Pancakes, waffles
• Chocolate (except some dark chocolate products)	• Salad dressings (ranch, blue cheese, creamy. Ceasar)
• Chowders	• Shakes
• Cocoa drinks, hot chocolate mixes	• Souffles
• Cream, sour cream, half & half, whipped cream, creamed or creamy foods	• Soups (esp. creamed)
• Custard, pudding	• Tuna (some canned tuna contains casein)
• Desserts	• Whey protein powder
• Flour Mixes	• Yogurt

Egg may also be listed as albumin, ovalbumin, ovo-mucoid, ovotransferrin, and lysozyme

Hidden sources of egg		
• Baby foods (some) • Baked goods • Batter mixes and battered foods • Bavarian Cream • Beers (some) • Boiled dressing • Bouillon • Breads and breaded foods (some), especially with shiny crusts • Cakes • Candy (some) • Cheese (some may have lysozyme as an unlabeled additive) • Coffee (some; to produce clarification) • Consommés • Cookies (some) Creamy fillings, cream puffs, creamed foods, creamed pies • Croquettes	• Custards • Doughnuts • Egg drop soup • Egg noodles • Egg rolls • Egg substitutes (some) • Eggnog • Flan • Flour mixes • Fondue • French toast • Fritters • Frosting • Glazed foods and baked goods • Hamburger mix • Hollandaise sauce • Ice cream • Macaroons • Malted drinks • Marshmallows • Mayonnaise • Meatloaf • Meringues	• Muffins (some) • Noodles (some) • Pancakes (most) • Pie fillings (some) • Powdered or dry eggs • Prepared meats (egg as a binding agent) • Pretzels (some) • Puddings • Quiche • Root beers (some; used to produce foam) • Salad dressings (some) • Sauces • Sausages • Sherbets • Soufflés • Soups (some) • Tartar sauce • Waffles • Wine (some; to produce clarification)

Soy

Forms of soy used in food products
• Soybeans AKA soya
• Soybean oil
• Soy lecithin
• Soy protein (concentrate, hydrolyzed, isolate)
• Soy (cheese, fiber, flour, grits, milk, nuts, yogurt, ice cream, pasta)
• Bean sprouts (soy)
• Edamame
• Kinako
• Miso
• Natto
• Nimame
• Okara
• Shoyu
• Soy sauce
• Tamari
• Tempeh
• Tofu (dofu, kori-dofu) AKA soybean curd
• Yuba
• Hydrolyzed soy protein (HSP)

Hidden Sources of Soy

• Asian Sauces (soy sauce, fish sauce, Pad Thai sauce, tempura sauce, ter-ryaki sauce) • Baby foods & formula	• Energy bars, nutrition bars, protein bars • Gravies	• Mixed tocopherols • Mono- and di-glycerides

• Baked goods and baking mixes (breads, biscuits, cakes, crackers, cereal, pastries) • Bouillon cubes & broths • Bulking agent • Butter substitute • Candy • Canned tuna (many contain textured vegetable protein; low- salt versions tend to be pure tuna with no fillers) • Cereal • Chicken broth, chicken processed with chicken broth • Chocolate	• Guar gum • Gum arabic • Hydrolyzed plant protein (HPP) or hydro-lyzed vegetable protein (HVP) • Ice Cream • Imitation dairy foods and milk substitutes (soy milk, vegan cheese) • Lecithin • Lunch/deli meats, prepared meats, meat products with fillers (such as burgers, sausages) • Margarine • Mayonnaise • Meat substitutes (veggie burg-ers, imitation chicken patties, imitation lunch meats, imitation bacon bits, imi-tation crab, etc)	• Natural flavoring • Nutrition supplements (vitamins) • Oil, Crisco spray • Pasta, noodles • Peanut but-ter and pea-nut butter substitutes • Protein powder • Salad Dressing • Smoothies • Soup • Stabilizer • Textured vegetable protein (TVP) • Thickener • Vegetable gum, starch, shortening, or oil • Vitamin E

Peanut Ingredients in Foods

• Arachis oil (another name for peanut oil) and peanut oil • Artificial nuts, beer nuts, ground nuts, mixed nuts, monkey nuts, nut meat, nut pieces • Cold-pressed, expelled or extruded pea-nut oil* • Goobers • Mandelonas (peanuts soaked in almond flavoring) • Peanut butter • Peanut flour • Peanut protein hydrolysate	• Candy • Chili • Egg rolls • Enchilada sauce • Glazes and marinades • Ice creams • Marzipan • Nougat • Pancakes • Salad dressing	• Sauces (chili sauce, hot sauce, pesto, gravy, mole sauce) • Specialty pizzas • Sweets such as pudding, cookies, baked goods, pies and hot chocolate • Vegetarian food products, especially meat substitutes

Food Substitutions

Listed below are suggested substitutions for foods that people commonly consume but often contain ingredients on the "Avoid" list. As more people are identifying food sensitivities, more products are coming out, so this is not a complete list.

Instead of:	Try:
Wheat bread	It is difficult to find a bread that is wheat-, corn-, dairy-, and egg-free, so check the ingredient list. If you are just eliminating one item, it may be possible to find breads that do not contain that (such as BFree bread, which is gluten-free and egg-free but contains corn)
Breading/ breadcrumbs	Grind rice crackers or use gluten-free breadcrumbs (check ingredients if doing the full elimination)
Wheat cereals	Certified gluten-free oats, cream of rice, puffed millet, puffed rice, crispy rice cereal, and homemade granola
Baking pow-der (contains cornstarch and often contains aluminum)	Hain Pure Foods Featherweight Baking Powder (contains potato starch) or mix your own: 1 tsp baking powder can be replaced by 1 ¼ tsp cream of tartar and ½ tsp baking soda
Corn oil	Non-GMO canola, coconut, olive, sun-flower, and safflower oils
Cornstarch	Potato, arrowroot, rice flours or starch
Cheese	Rice and almond cheeses—read labels and look for casein-free

Chips	Kale chips (Trader Joe's has a Zesty Nacho flavor), seaweed snacks, veggie chips (make sure if it is processed that there is no added wheat), roasted and salted vegetables (read ingredients to make sure no corn oil or dextrin)
Crackers	Rice cakes, rice crackers, Nut-Thins (from pecan, almond, and rice)
Eggs	Ener-G egg replacer; blend 1 Tablespoon of flax seeds in blender with ¼ cup water and allow to thicken
Ice cream	Rice Dream Coconut Ice Cream; 100% frozen fruit juice bars or berry sorbets (watch sugar content!)
Jelly/jam	All-fruit jam (no added sugar or other sweetener)
Pasta	Quinoa pasta; rice noodles; 100% buckwheat udon or soba noodles; sweet potato vermicelli (dang myun); Japanese shirataki noodles; kelp noodles; spiralized zucchini; spaghetti squash; cellophane noodles, glass noodles, bean vermicelli, or bean threads
Peanut butter	Other nut/seed butters (almond, sunflower, sesame)
Soda	Water, water with lemon, lime, mint or fruit; herbal tea; seltzer and juice; diluted fruit juice; vegetable juice
Soy Sauce	Coconut aminos
Sugar	Maple syrup, blackstrap molasses, green leaf stevia (check ingredients and avoid if there are other added sweeteners), honey

Wheat and wheat flour	Almond and other nut meals/flours, amaranth, arrowroot flour buckwheat, bean flours: Chickpea (Garbanzo), fava, romano, garfava (garbanzo and fava) flour, coconut flour, flaxmeal, legumes (beans, peas, lentils), mesquite flour, millet, montina flour, oats that are certified gluten-free, pea flour, potato flour, quinoa, rice, sorghum Starchy vegetables (potatoes, carrots, parsnips, pumpkin, squash, yams and sweet potatoes), tapioca (manioc, cassava, yucca), teff. 1 cup wheat flour is equivalent to: 7/8 cup rice flour ½ cup arrowroot starch 5/8 cup potato starch flour ¾ cup tapioca starch 1 cup teff flour 1 tablespoon flour for thickening sauces or gravies equals: ½ tablespoon potato, tapioca, rice, or arrowroot starch.
Wheat/corn Tortillas	Rice tortilla, teff tortilla, paleo wrap, coconut wrap

Appendix B: Meal Plan and Recipes

Sample 7-Day Meal Plan

Day 1	
Breakfast	Easy Beans and Greens
Snack	Hummus and fresh vegetable crudité
Lunch	Brown Rice and Black Bean Bowl
Snack	Almond butter on apples
Dinner	Baked Salmon with Dill with quinoa and broccoli
Day 2	
Breakfast	Chia Breakfast Pudding
Snack	Sliced turkey and avocado rolled in spinach leaves
Lunch	Sautéed Kale with Cannellini Beans
Snack	Kale chips with guacamole
Dinner	Simple Baked Chicken Drumsticks with Cilantro Lime Cauliflower Rice and salad
Day 3	
Breakfast	Basic Breakfast Smoothie
Snack	Sunflower butter on celery
Lunch	Stir-Fry Vegetables with Chicken and brown rice
Snack	Hummus and rice crackers
Dinner	Broiled Lamb Chops with Rosemary, quinoa, and Leafy Greens with Red Onions and Raisins

Day 4	
Breakfast	Apple Cinnamon Breakfast Quinoa
Snack	Green drink
Lunch	Buckwheat noodle salad
Snack	Coconut yogurt with granola and fresh berries
Dinner	Walnut-Crusted Fish, Quinoa, and Roasted Vegetables
Day 5	
Breakfast	Breakfast Hash
Snack	Fruit salad
Lunch	Collard Wraps
Snack	Kale chips with guacamole
Dinner	Spaghetti Squash with Tomato Sauce, Sesame Brussels Sprouts Sauté
Day 6	
Breakfast	Coconut yogurt with granola and fresh berries
Snack	Hummus and rice crackers
Lunch	Lentil and Split Pea Soup
Snack	Protein bar
Dinner	Baked Chicken with Cabbage, Carrots, and Onions
Day 7	
Breakfast	Basic Breakfast Smoothie
Snack	Lentil and Split Pea Soup
Lunch	Thai Quinoa Bowl
Snack	Almond butter on celery
Dinner	Korean Chap Chae Noodles, Korean-Style Mung Bean Sprouts, and brown rice

All included recipes are gluten-free, dairy-free, soy-free, egg-free, corn-free, and peanut-free.

Breakfasts
Basic Breakfast Smoothie
Servings: 1 Prep time: 5 minutes Cook time: 0 minutes

- 1 cup liquid (water, coconut water, or rice milk)
- 1 scoop pea, hemp, or rice protein powder
- 1 tablespoon flax seed, chia seed, or hemp seed
- ½ to 1 cup berries (raspberry, blueberry, or strawberry)
- ¼ to 1 cup spinach, kale, or other leafy green
- Optional: ¼ avocado or ¼ cup nuts soaked overnight
- Optional: 1 tablespoon coconut or flaxseed oil

Choose your favorite ingredients and combine in a blender.

Easy Beans and Greens
Servings: 1 Prep time: 5 minutes Cook time: 5 minutes

- ½ to 1 cup beans (pinto, cannellini, or black), soaked overnight and cooked or rinsed canned beans
- 2 tablespoons salsa fresca
- 1 cup chopped greens (kale or baby spinach)
- Optional: salt, pepper, cumin

Heat the beans in a skillet on medium heat until warm. Add the salsa and chopped greens and heat until wilted. Season with salt, pepper, and cumin to taste.

Apple Cinnamon Breakfast Quinoa
Servings: 4 Prep time: 5 minutes Cook time: 20 minutes

- 1 cup dry quinoa, rinsed well
- 1 ½ cups water
- 1 teaspoon cinnamon, plus more for sprinkling
- 2 teaspoons real vanilla extract
- ½ cup unsweetened applesauce

- ¼ cup golden raisins
- 1 cup warmed rice, almond, or coconut milk
- 1 gala apple, peeled and diced
- 1 to 2 tablespoons chia seeds, hemp seeds, or ground flaxseed

Combine quinoa, water, cinnamon, and vanilla in a small saucepan and bring to a boil. Reduce to a simmer, cover, and let cook for 15 minutes, or until quinoa can be fluffed with a fork. Divide the cooked quinoa into four servings then stir in applesauce, raisins, and warmed milk substitute. Top with fresh cut apples, chia seeds, and a dash of cinnamon.

Chia Breakfast Pudding

Servings: 1 Prep time: 5 minutes Cook time: Overnight to sit

- 1 tablespoon chia seeds
- 1 cup almond, rice, or hemp milk
- ¼ cup frozen berries
- ½ to 1 tablespoon maple syrup (optional)

Combine all ingredients and mix well. Store overnight in the refrigerator and enjoy in the morning. (I prefer to put all of the ingredients in a mason jar.)

Breakfast Hash

Servings: 2 Prep time: 10 minutes Cook time: 20 minutes

- 1 tablespoon coconut oil
- 1 onion, diced
- 3 garlic cloves, diced
- 1 medium sweet potato, shredded
- Chicken or vegetable broth, if needed
- 1 bunch dino kale, chopped roughly

- Your choice of organic and preservative-free meat, diced (optional)
- Other cooked veggies (such as roasted Brussels sprouts or parsnips) (optional)
- ¼ avocado, sliced (optional)

Heat a skillet over medium-high heat. If cooking meat, cook fully and remove from the pan, setting it aside. Add the coconut oil to the pan until hot. Add the onion and garlic and sauté until translucent. Add the sweet potato and cook about 5 minutes more. Add more coconut oil, if needed, or deglaze with broth. Add the kale and cook until just wilted. If using meat or other cooked veggies, add to the pan and toss everything together. Top with sliced avocado if desired.

Easy Gluten-Free Granola
Servings: 8 Prep time: 5 minutes Cook time: 25 minutes

- 3 cups gluten-free rolled oats
- 1 cup unsweetened coconut chips
- ¼ cup coconut oil, melted
- 1/3 cup maple syrup
- ½ teaspoon cinnamon
- ½ teaspoon real vanilla extract
- Pinch sea salt
- 1 teaspoon chia seeds (optional)

Preheat the oven to 350 degrees Fahrenheit. In a large mixing bowl, combine the oats and coconut chips. In a small bowl, combine the coconut oil, maple syrup, cinnamon, vanilla, and salt, and add to the oat mixture. Stir well to fully coat the oats. Spread evenly on a cookie sheet and bake for 10 minutes. Remove from the oven to stir, then place back into the oven for another 10 minutes. Remove from the oven to stir a second time, then place back into the oven for 5 more minutes. Turn off the oven and let cool.

Spaghetti Squash Hash Browns

Servings: 2 Prep time: 10 minutes Cook time: 20 minutes

- 1 tablespoon oil
- 2 cups cooked and shredded spaghetti squash (about ½ of a small cooked squash)

Heat the oil in a large skillet over medium heat. Press the water out of the squash with paper towels. Form little patties by pressing about 2 tablespoons of the squash firmly between your palms. Place the patties gently on the warmed skillet and cook 5 to 7 minutes per side. Transfer to paper towels to drain. Serve warm.

Snacks

Hummus and fresh vegetables or rice crackers
Almond butter or sunflower butter on carrots, apples, or celery
Sliced turkey and avocado rolled in spinach leaves
Kale chips with guacamole
Green drink
Fruit salad
Read labels, of course, but these brands have some bars that are gluten-/soy-/dairy-/egg-free: Rise Energy Bar, Amazing Grass Green Superfood, Organic Food Bar, Pure Bar, and Larabar

Hummus

Servings: 8 Prep time: 15 minutes Cook time: 0 minutes

- 2 (15-ounce) cans of chickpeas, rinsed and drained (or 3 ½ cups cooked chickpeas)
- 6 tablespoons sesame tahini
- 6 tablespoons fresh lemon juice

- 1 teaspoon minced garlic
- 1 teaspoon ground cumin
- 1 teaspoon cayenne
- ½ teaspoon salt
- extra-virgin olive oil, for drizzling

Place all ingredients except cayenne and olive oil in a blender or food processor and purée to a thick paste. Add the cayenne and salt. Transfer to a container with a tight-fitting lid and smooth the top. Pour olive oil on top and tilt until it coats the surface. Cover and refrigerate until use.

Green Drink
Servings: 1 Prep time: 15 minutes Cook time: 0 minutes

- 2 handfuls of kale, spinach, romaine
- 1 to 2 stalks celery
- 1 medium cucumber
- 1 medium apple
- ½ inch slice of peeled fresh ginger root

In a high-speed blender or juicer, combine all the ingredients and blend until smooth.

Lunches and Dinner
Rice/quinoa/millet/starchy vegetables with baked/grilled/broiled lean protein and veggies (steamed, stir-fried, roasted, or sautéed) are always a great option.

Easy Salad Dressing
Servings: 2 Prep time: 5 minutes Cook time: 0 minutes

- 1 ½ tablespoons fresh lemon juice
- 1 ½ tablespoons extra-virgin olive oil
- ¼ teaspoon freshly ground black pepper

- 1/8 teaspoon kosher salt

Combine lemon juice, olive oil, black pepper, and salt in a large bowl, and stir with a whisk.

Brown Rice and Black Bean Bowl

Servings: 4 Prep time: 10 minutes Cook time: 20 minutes

- 2 tablespoons coconut oil
- 2 cups chopped organic baby spinach
- 2 cups cooked brown rice
- 2 cups black beans, soaked overnight and cooked, or rinsed canned beans
- 1 teaspoon sea salt
- 1 teaspoon garlic powder
- 1 teaspoon cumin
- 1 avocado, chopped
- 1 cup chopped tomatoes

Heat a large pan over medium-high heat. Add the coconut oil to the pan and heat. Add the spinach and sauté until just wilted. Add the rice, beans, sea salt, garlic powder, and cumin. Cook until all ingredients are heated through. Remove from heat. Before serving, gently fold in avocado and tomatoes.

Buckwheat Noodle Salad

Servings: 4 Prep time: 20 minutes Cook time: 25 minutes

- ¼ cup, plus 2 tablespoons rice vinegar
- 1 teaspoon sugar
- 2 tablespoons peeled and finely grated fresh ginger
- 1 tablespoon honey
- 2 tablespoons coconut aminos
- 2 teaspoons toasted sesame oil
- 2 teaspoons chili sauce

- ¼ cup organic canola oil
- 12 ounces buckwheat noodles, cooked according to package directions, rinsed under cold water and drained
- 1 carrot, peeled and shredded
- 1 organic red bell pepper, seeded and julienned
- ¼ organic English cucumber, peeled and grated
- 3 green onions, thinly sliced
- ¼ cup chopped fresh cilantro leaves

In a large bowl, whisk together the rice vinegar, sugar, ginger, honey, coconut aminos, sesame oil, and chili sauce until combined. Slowly whisk in the canola oil until the dressing is emulsified. Add the remaining ingredients. Gently mix to combine and serve.

Collard Wraps
Servings: 4 Prep time: 20 minutes Cook time: 0 minutes

- 4 large collard leaves
- Juice of ½ lemon
- 1 cup raw pecans
- 1 tablespoon coconut aminos
- 1 teaspoon cumin
- 1 teaspoon extra-virgin olive oil
- 1 organic red bell pepper, sliced
- 1 avocado, sliced
- Juice of ½ lime
- 2 to 3 ounces organic alfalfa sprouts

Wash the collard leaves, cut off the white stem at the bottom, and place in a bath of warm water with juice of half of a lemon. Let soak for 10 minutes, then dry the leaves with a paper towel. Using a knife, make a thin slice down the central root but do not cut the leaf in half. This makes it easier to bend the leaves while wrapping. In a food processor, combine the pecans, coconut aminos, cumin, and olive oil. Pulse until combined and mixture clumps together. Place a collard leaf on your work surface and spread the nut mix, then layer red pepper slices, avocado slices, a drizzle of lime juice, and alfafa sprouts. Fold over the top and bottom and then wrap up the sides. Slice in half and serve.

Cilantro Lime Cauliflower Rice
Servings: 6 Prep time: 15 minutes Cook time: 15 minutes

- 1 head cauliflower (about 6 cups or 24 ounces chopped)
- 1 tablespoon extra-virgin olive oil
- 2 garlic cloves
- 2 scallions, diced
- ¼ teaspoon sea salt
- ¼ teaspoon freshly ground black pepper
- 3 tablespoons fresh lime juice
- ¼ cups fresh, chopped cilantro

Rinse cauliflower, and pat dry. Chop into florets, and grate in a food processor until it resembles the size of rice or couscous. Heat a large pan over medium heat, and add olive oil, garlic, and scallions. Sauté for 3 to 4 minutes. Increase the heat to medium-high, and add the cauliflower. Sauté for 5 to 6 minutes more. Remove from heat and transfer to a large bowl (before cauliflower gets mushy). Toss with the sea salt, black pepper, lime juice, and cilantro.

Roasted Vegetables
Servings: 4 Prep time: 5 minutes Cook time: 20 minutes

- 1 pound assorted vegetables (such as carrots, asparagus, and sugar snap peas)
- 4 unpeeled garlic cloves
- 2 tablespoons extra-virgin olive oil

- Kosher salt
- Freshly ground pepper

Preheat oven to 450 degrees Fahrenheit. Combine the vegetables, garlic, and olive oil in a large bowl. Season with the salt and black pepper. Toss to coat. Spread the vegetables in a single layer on a baking sheet. Roast until tender, stirring halfway through, about 20 minutes.

Lentil and Split Pea Soup

Servings: 8 Prep time: 15 minutes Cook time: 1 hour

- 1 cup split peas, rinsed well
- 1 cup lentils, rinsed well
- 10 cups organic low-sodium vegetable broth
- 2 medium carrots, sliced
- 2 stalks organic celery, sliced
- 1 large organic red bell pepper, chopped
- 1 large onion, chopped
- 1 bay leaf
- 1 teaspoon cumin
- ¼ teaspoon ground black pepper
- ½ teaspoon salt

Put all the ingredients in a large pot and cook for 1 hour, stirring occasionally. Remove the bay leaf before serving.

Korean Chap Chae Noodles

Servings: 4 Prep time: 20 minutes Cook time: 20 minutes

- 3 tablespoons organic canola oil, divided
- 2 cups julienned carrots
- Kosher salt, to taste
- Freshly ground white pepper, to taste
- 2 cups thinly sliced onions

- 1 cup julienned organic red bell pepper
- 1 garlic clove, minced
- 1/3 cup coconut aminos
- 1 tablespoon sugar
- 16 ounces dried Korean sweet potato noodles (dangmyeon), cooked according to package directions, rinsed with cold water and drained
- 2 tablespoons toasted sesame oil
- 2 tablespoons thinly sliced scallion
- 1 tablespoon toasted sesame seeds

Heat 1 tablespoon of canola oil in a large skillet over medium-high heat. Add the carrots and season with salt and pepper. Cook, stirring, until half-tender, about 3 minutes. Transfer the carrots to a large bowl. Heat 1 tablespoon of canola oil and cook the onions, pepper, and garlic until just tender, about 5 minutes. Meanwhile mix together coconut aminos and sugar in a small bowl and add to the onion and peppers for the last minute to dissolve the sugar. Transfer the mixture to the bowl with carrots, add cooked noodles and sesame oil, and toss. Garnish with scallions and sesame seeds.

Korean-Style Seasoned Mung Bean Sprouts
Servings: 4 Prep time: 5 minutes Cook time: 10 minutes

- 12 ounces fresh mung bean sprouts
- 6 cups water
- 1 teaspoon plus ½ teaspoon salt
- 1 teaspoon thinly sliced scallion
- ½ teaspoon minced garlic
- 1 teaspoon roasted sesame seeds
- 1 tablespoon toasted sesame oil

Rinse the mung bean sprouts in cold water. Boil the water in a pot and add 1 teaspoon of salt. Once the water starts to boil, plunge the bean sprouts into the pot and allow them to cook for 1 to 2 minutes. Drain the water and rinse the sprouts with cold water for 1 minute. Squeeze the bean sprouts with your hands to remove excess water and put them into a bowl. Add the scallion, garlic, sesame seeds, sesame oil, and ½ teaspoon salt and mix well.

Thai Quinoa Bowl
Servings: 2 Prep time: 15 minutes Cook time: 20 minutes

For the bowl:
- ½ cup quinoa, cooked according to package directions
- ½ cup steamed broccoli florets or kale
- ½ cup cooked butternut squash or sweet potato, cut into bite-sized chunks
- ¼ cup chopped scallion
- ¼ cup chopped cilantro

For the dressing:
- Juice of ½ a lime
- 1 teaspoon sesame seeds
- 1 tablespoon coconut aminos
- 1 tablespoon sesame oil
- 1 tablespoon rice vinegar
- 2 garlic cloves, minced

In a large bowl toss the cooked quinoa, broccoli, butternut squash, scallion, and cilantro. Mix until combined. In a small bowl combine dressing ingredients. Pour the dressing over quinoa and mix until combined.

Broccoli with Garlic
Servings: 4 Prep time: 5 minutes Cook time: 6 minutes

- ½ cup water
- 1 pound broccoli, cut into florets

- 2 to 3 tablespoons extra-virgin olive oil
- 1 teaspoon minced or crushed garlic
- Salt
- Freshly ground black pepper
- Red pepper flakes (optional)

Add ½ cup of water to a large pan and heat over medium-high heat. Add the broccoli florets and cover, allowing to steam for 2 to 3 minutes until broccoli is bright green. Drizzle the olive oil over the broccoli and stir in the garlic, cooking for another 2 to 3 minutes. Add the salt and pepper to taste, and sprinkle with the red pepper flakes if desired.

Sautéed Kale with Cannellini Beans

Servings: 4 Prep time: 15 minutes Cook time: 10 minutes

- 2 tablespoons extra-virgin olive oil
- 1 red onion, peeled and sliced thin
- 4 garlic cloves, minced
- 2 bunches kale, chopped
- 2 tablespoons mirin
- 3 cups cooked cannellini beans, rinsed
- Salt and pepper to taste

In a large pot over medium heat, heat the olive oil. Add the onion and garlic and sauté until soft, about 3 minutes. Add the kale and mirin and sauté 4 to 5 minutes or until kale is bright green and tender. Add the beans and sauté 2 minutes to heat through. Remove from heat, season with salt and pepper to taste.

Quinoa

Servings: 4 Prep time: 5 to 60 minutes Cook time: 15 minutes

- 1 cup quinoa
- 1 ½ cups water or stock
- Thumb-size piece of kombu or pinch of sea salt
- Seasonings to taste: salt, pepper, oregano, basil, parsley, olive oil

If you have time, add the quinoa to a pot with enough water to cover and soak for at least 1 hour. Then strain and rinse.

Place the quinoa in a pot, add the fresh water or stock and the kombu or salt, and bring to a boil. Reduce heat to simmer, cover, and cook until all liquid is absorbed, about 15 minutes. Remove from heat, discard kombu, fluff with a fork, and serve. Season to taste, if desired.

Garlic-Sesame Brussels Sprouts

Servings: 4 Prep time: 10 minutes Cook time: 20 minutes

- 2 tablespoons extra-virgin olive oil
- 2 garlic cloves, minced
- 2 cups Brussels sprouts, trimmed and sliced in half
- 1 tablespoon mirin
- Water as needed
- 1 tablespoon toasted sesame oil
- ¼ cup toasted sesame seeds
- Salt to taste

Heat olive oil in a large skillet over medium heat. Sauté garlic until soft, about 1 minute. Add the Brussels sprouts and mirin and sauté for 15 minutes. If sprouts stick to the skillet or start to char, add a tablespoon of water to deglaze the pan. Repeat as needed. Once cooked, remove from heat, then toss with the toasted sesame oil and sesame seeds. Season to taste with salt.

Spaghetti Squash with Tomato Sauce
Servings: 4 Prep time: 10 minutes Cook time: 60 minutes

- 1 spaghetti squash
- 1 tablespoon extra-virgin olive oil
- 1 garlic clove, minced
- ½ onion, chopped
- 1 medium zucchini, cut into half-rounds about ¼ inch thick
- 1 medium organic bell pepper, chopped
- 1 (15-ounce) can diced tomatoes
- ½ teaspoon dried oregano
- ½ teaspoon dried basil
- Salt and pepper to taste

Preheat oven to 400 degrees Fahrenheit. Place the squash on cookie sheet, pierce a few times with a knife, and bake 1 hour or until soft. Remove from the oven and set aside. While the squash is cooking, heat the olive oil in a saucepan over medium-low heat, add the garlic, and sauté for 1 to 2 minutes. Add the onion, zucchini, and pepper and cook 3 to 4 minutes, stirring occasionally. Add the diced tomatoes, oregano, and basil, and simmer on low heat until the squash is finished. Cut the squash in half lengthwise and remove and discard seeds. Hold half of the squash over a serving bowl and, using a fork, scrape out the flesh from top to bottom to separate the strands of squash. Repeat with the other half. Top with the tomato sauce and serve.

Leafy Greens with Red Onions and Raisins
Servings: 4 Prep time: 5 minutes Cook time: 15 minutes

- 2 tablespoons extra-virgin olive oil
- 1 red onion, cut into quarters
- Sea salt

- 1 garlic clove, minced
- 1/3 cup raisins
- Water as needed
- 1 bunch organic kale or Swiss chard, rinsed, stemmed, and chopped

In a large sauté pan, heat the olive oil over medium-high heat. Add the onions and a pinch of salt and sauté for 3 to 5 minutes. Add the garlic and stir for about 30 seconds. Add the raisins and stir for about 30 seconds more. Add the greens one handful at a time to the pan until the pan is full. Add a pinch of salt and cook until bright green and tender, about 2 to 3 minutes. If needed, add a tablespoon of water and cover the pan, cooking for an additional 2 to 3 minutes.

Stir-Fry Vegetables with Chicken

Servings 4 Prep time: 15 minutes Cook time: 15 minutes

- 2 tablespoons organic canola oil, divided
- 1 pound boneless organic chicken breasts, cut into bite-sized chunks
- 2 garlic cloves, minced
- 1 tablespoon grated fresh ginger
- Water as needed
- 1 cup broccoli florets
- 3 carrots, julienned
- 1 organic red pepper, julienned
- 2 scallions, chopped
- 1 tablespoon coconut aminos

Heat a skillet over medium-high heat. Add 1 tablespoon of the canola oil to the pan. Add the chicken to the pan, stirring occasionally, until it starts to brown, about 7 to 8 minutes. Remove the chicken from the pan and keep in a covered container. Add the remaining tablespoon of canola oil to the pan. Cook the garlic and ginger for 1 minute, adding a small amount of water to the pan if anything starts to stick. Add the broccoli and carrots and cook for 2 to 3 minutes, stirring occasionally. Stir in the red pepper, scallions, and coconut aminos, and cook 1 minute longer.

Note: <u>Chicken can be omitted for vegetarian version.</u>

Walnut-Crusted Fish

Servings: 4 Prep time: 20 minutes Cook time: 10 minutes

- 4 4-ounce flounder, sole, or tilapia fillets
- ¼ cup almond milk
- 1 cup finely chopped walnuts
- ¼ teaspoon salt
- ¼ teaspoon freshly ground black pepper
- 1 ½ tablespoons extra-virgin olive oil
- 1 tablespoon fresh lemon juice
- ¼ cup chopped fresh parsley for garnish

Rinse the fish in cold water and pat dry with paper towel. Place the almond milk in a shallow bowl. Spread the chopped walnuts, salt, and pepper on a plate. Dip the fish in the almond milk and then dredge in the walnut mixture, gently pressing the walnuts onto the fish to form the crust. Heat a large skillet over medium heat. Add the olive oil and heat until it shimmers, then add the fish. Cook for 3 to 4 minutes on each side, until the fish is cooked through. Squeeze the lemon juice over the top, then sprinkle with the parsley.

Simple Baked Chicken Drumsticks

Servings: 4 Prep time: 5 minutes Cook time: 1 hour

- Extra-virgin olive oil
- 5 to 6 organic chicken drumsticks

- Garlic powder
- Freshly ground black pepper
- Salt

Preheat oven to 375 degrees Fahrenheit. Coat the bottom of a 9 X 13 baking pan with the olive oil. Add drumsticks. Sprinkle generously with the garlic powder and black pepper. Sprinkle lightly with the salt. Bake for 30 minutes. Turn the drumsticks over and add more garlic powder, pepper, and salt. Bake another 30 minutes or until fully cooked.

Baked Chicken with Cabbage, Carrots, and Onions
Servings: 4 Prep time: 15 minutes Cook time: 50 minutes

- 4 organic chicken breast halves (skin-on)
- 1 head cabbage, chopped
- 1 large onion, peels and cut into eighths
- 1 pound carrots
- 1 teaspoon kosher salt, divided
- 1 teaspoon freshly ground black pepper, divided
- 2 to 3 teaspoons finely minced fresh rosemary
- 4 to 5 teaspoons minced garlic or 6 to 7 garlic cloves
- 1 lemon, quartered
- ¼ cup extra-virgin olive oil
- 3 tablespoons red wine vinegar

Preheat oven to 450 degrees Fahrenheit. Place the chicken, cabbage, onion, and carrots in a 9 by 13 baking pan. In a small bowl, mix together ½ teaspoon salt, ½ teaspoon pepper, and minced rosemary. Pour over the chicken and veggies and toss well. Arrange the chicken so that it lies on top of the veggies, skin-side up. Add the garlic and quartered lemon on top of veggies. In another small bowl, whisk together the olive oil, vinegar and remaining salt and pepper and drizzle over the chicken and veggies. Roast in the oven for 50 minutes until chicken is cooked through and vegetables are tender.

Baked Salmon with Dill

Servings: 4 Prep time: 5 minutes Cook time: 15 minutes

- 4 (5-ounce) wild-caught salmon fillets
- 4 teaspoons extra-virgin olive oil
- 4 teaspoons chopped fresh dill
- ¼ teaspoon salt
- ¼ teaspoon freshly ground black pepper

Preheat oven to 375 degrees Fahrenheit. Line a cookie sheet with parchment paper or oil the pan. Add the salmon to the pan. Mix together the olive oil, dill, salt, and black pepper, and brush over the salmon. Bake for 12 to 15 minutes.

Broiled Lamb Chops with Rosemary

Servings: 4 Prep time: 5 minutes Cook time: 15 minutes

- 2 teaspoons extra-virgin olive oil
- 4 lamb chops
- 1 teaspoon dried rosemary
- 1 tablespoon fresh rosemary
- ½ teaspoon sea salt
- ½ teaspoon freshly ground black pepper

Preheat the broiler. Drizzle the olive oil over the lamb chops and rub to coat them. In a small bowl, mix together the rosemary, salt, and black pepper, and season both sides of the lamb chops. Place the lamb in a broiler pan and broil for 8 to 10 minutes, turning once during cooking. When done, the lamb should be only slightly pink in the center.

Chocolate Chip Cookie Dough Bites

Servings: 10 Prep time: 15 minutes Cook time: 0 minutes

- 2/3 cup raw cashews
- 1/3 cup gluten-free oats
- Pinch of sea salt
- 1 vanilla bean or 1 ½ teaspoons of vanilla extract
- 2 tablespoons pure maple syrup
- 1 tablespoon honey
- 1 teaspoon coconut oil (optional)
- High-quality dark chocolate chips, at least 60% cacao

*you can add Maca powder, chia seeds, powdered greens, flax, or hemp seeds to "superfood-ize" these.

Put the cashews and oats in blender or food processor and blend to a fine meal. Add the rest of the ingredients except the chocolate chips and blend until a nice dough consistency forms. Stir in the chocolate chips. If dough is too sticky, place in fridge for 10 to 15 minutes. Put the dough on a work surface and take a tablespoon of dough at a time and roll into little cookie bites. Refrigerate or freeze.

Appendix C: Resources

For more information on what I do and to find additional resources, see valenciaporter.com. Items mentioned specifically may be found below.

Chapter 3:
Healthcare Providers Knowledgeable in Environmental Medicine

- American Academy of Environmental Medicine: aaemonline.org/find.php
- Dr. Crinnion's Comprehensive Training in Environmental Medicine: crinnionopinion.com/doctors-who-have-completed-this-training
- Functional Medicine Fellowship: ifm.org/find-a-practitioner
- Integrative Medicine Fellowship: integrativemedicine.arizona.edu/alumni.html

Lab Testing

- Genova Diagnostics: Toxic Core Panel, Functional Nutrient, Genetic Testing: gdx.net
- Doctor's Data: Heavy Metal Pre- and Post-Chelation: doctorsdata.com
- Realtime Laboratories: Urine Mold Mycotoxins: realtimelab.com

- Great Plains Laboratories: Organic Acids, Glyphosate, Urine Mold Mycotoxins, Toxic Nonmetal Profile, Glyphosate: greatplainslaboratory.com
- Spectracell: Functional Nutrient Testing, Thyroid and Hormone Testing: spectracell.com
- 23andMe: Genetic Testing (but must analyze the raw data through another service): 23andme.com
- Pathway Genomics: Genetic Testing: pathway.com

Chapter 4:
Ayurvedic Practitioners and Training Courses
- Chopra Center for Wellbeing: chopra.com
- National Ayurvedic Medical Association: ayurvedanama.org
- Ayurvedic Institute: ayurveda.com
- Kerala Ayurveda: ayurvedaacademy.com

Chapter 5:
2. Organic Foods and Pesticides
- EWG'S Shopper's Guide to Pesticides in Produce: ewg.org/foodnews
- To find local Community Supported Agriculture (CSA): localharvest.org/csa
- Pesticide Action Network: panna.org

3. Non-GMO foods and Glyphosate
- Glyphosate Testing: detoxproject.org, greatplainslaboratory.com, hrilabs.org/glyphosate-testing/
- UCSD Herbicide Awareness and Research Project
- Non-GMO Foods: livingnongmo.org
- Ratings for Nutrition, Ingredients, and Processing: ewg.org/foodscores

4. Plant-Based Diet
- Forks Over Knives: forksoverknives.com

- The 30-Day Vegan Challenge: 30dayveganchallenge.com
- Eat for the Planet: onegreenplanet.org/eatfortheplanet

5. Choosing Safer Fish
- NRDC's Smart Seafood Buying Guide: nrdc.org/stories/ smart-seafood-buying-guide
- EWG's Consumers Guide to Seafood: ewg.org/research/ ewgs-good-seafood-guide
- Monterey Bay Seafood Watch: seafoodwatch.org
- Vital Choice Wild Seafood and Organics: vitalchoice. com/?idaffiliate=504244

6. Clean Water
- EWG's Tap Water Database: ewg.org/tapwater
- EWG's Water Filter Guide: ewg.org/tapwater/water-filter-guide.php
- Searchable Annual Drinking Water Report: ofmpub. epa.gov/apex/safewater/f?p=136:102:::NO:RP,102::
- Certified Laboratories for Drinking Water Testing: epa.gov/dwlabcert/contact-information-certification-programs-and-certified-laboratories-drinking-water
- Earth Justice Advocacy Campaign to Fight Fracking: earthjustice.org/advocacy-campaigns/unfracktured

9. Fiber and Bowel Movements
- Find a Colon Hydrotherapist: i-act.org/IACTSearch. HTM
- Triphala, Probiotics, FiberMend by Thorne: valencia-porter.com/supplements

10. Liver Support
- For Supplements: valenciaporter.com/supplements

11. Tea sources
- Mountain Rose Herbs

- Numi Organic
- Yogic
- Traditional Medicinals
- Zhena's Gypsy Tea
- Tea Leaf Co
- Rishi Tea
- Choice Organic
- Mighty Leaf
- Pukka Tea

14. Plastic

- #Crushplastic Movement for Plastic Alternatives: one-greenplanet.org/crushplastic/
- BPA-free Brands: Eden, Amy's, Annie's Organic, Sprouts Farmers Market, Muir Glen

15. Ayurvedic Nutrition

- *Food as Medicine* by Todd Caldecott
- *Ayurvedic Cooking for Self-Healing* by Usha Lad and Vasant Lad
- *The Tastes of Ayurveda* and *The Modern Ayurvedic Cookbook* by Amrita Sondhi

Chapter 6:

17. Gene Testing

- 23andMe: 23andme.com
- Pathway Genomics: pathway.com

18. Nurture Your Inner Garden

- Probiotics: valenciaporter.com/supplements
- Microbiome Testing
  - Genova Diagnostics: GI Effects, SIBO Breath test: gdx.net
  - Viome: www.viome.com/?rfsn=814854.977687

19. Personal Care Products & Cosmetics
- Skin Deep database: ewg.org/skindeep
- Campaign for Safe Cosmetics: safecosmetics.org
- Made Safe certification: madesafe.org

20. Sunscreens
- EWG's Annual Sunscreen Guide: ewg.org/sunscreen

26. Breathe
- Demonstration of breathing techniques at: valencia-porter.com/breathe

27. Sauna
- Clearlight: infraredsauna.com
- Heavenly Heat: heavenlyheatsaunas.com
- SaunaRay: saunaray.com
- Portable Units:
  - Saunaspace: saunaspace.com
  - SaunaFix: creatrixsolutions.com/sauna-fix

Chapter 7:
30. Green Your Cleaning Supplies
- EWG's Guide to Healthy Cleaning: ewg.org/guides/cleaners
- Labels to look for:
  - EPA SaferChoice: epa.gov/saferchoice and cleangredients.org
  - UL Ecologo: ul.com/environment
  - GreenSeal: greenseal.org
  - Made Safe certification: madesafe.org

31. Care for Your Air
- For resources and to find professionals Indoor Air Quality Association: iaqa.org
- Home Air Purifiers/Filters

- ○ IQ Air: iqair.com
- ○ BlueAir: blueair.com
- ○ Austin Air: austinair.com
- Car Air Filters
  - ○ aireox.com/model22d.html
  - ○ foustco.com/airpurifiers.html

33. Fire the Flame Retardants
- To send in a sample of polyurethane foam to Duke University to test for 7 different flame retardants: foam.pratt.duke.edu

34. Healthy Mattress Options
- My Green Mattress: mygreenmattress.com
- Sleep on Latex: sleeponlatex.com
- Samina Mattress: samina.com

37. EMF Protection
- Meters, Shielding products: lessemf.com

38. PVC-Free Toys, School Supplies, and Building Materials
- SafBaby: safbaby.com/lead-free-pvc-free-and-fire-retardant-free-toy-manufacturers
- Center for Health, Environment & Justice: chej.org/publications/PVCGuide/PVCfree.pdf
- Green Building Supply: greenbuildingsupply.com

40. Don't Live in a Moldy Home
- Mold Testing
  - ○ Urine mycotoxins test: Realtime Labs (realtimelab.com), Great Plains Lab: (greatplainslaboratory.com)
  - ○ HERTSMI and ERMI home/office mold test: Mycometrics.com
  - ○ Indoor Air Quality Association: iaqa.org
- Biotoxin/Mold Illness: survivingmold.com

41. Get the Lead Out
- IAOMT Safe Mercury Amalgam Removal Technique: iaomt.org/safe-removal-amalgam-fillings

43. Rethink Your Pest Control
- Integrated Pest Management: EcoWise, GreenPro, GreenShield
- Pesticide Action Network: Panna.org

Chapter 8
48. Practice Meditation or Mindfulness
- So Hum Guided Meditation: valenciaporter.com/media
- Chopra Center online meditation course: chopra.com/online-courses/primordial-sound-meditation/on-demand
- Guided meditations: davidji.com
- Apps: Headspace, Insight Timer, Inner Balance, and The Mindfulness App are some of my favorites

49. Forgiveness and Gratitude
- *Forgive For Good* by Fred Luskin
- *Free to Love, Free to Heal* by David Simon, M.D.

Chapter 9
50. Reduce, Reuse, Recycle
- OhmConnect app: ohmconnect.com

52. Karma of Consciousness
Prosperity Resources: well.org/prosperity/resources

Selected References

Baker, N. *The Body Toxic: How the Hazardous Chemistry of Everyday Things Threatens Our Health and Well-being*, North Point Press, 2009.

Carson, R. *Silent Spring*, Houghton Mifflin, 2002.

Crinnion, W. *Clean, Green, and Lean: Get Rid of the Toxins That Make You Fat*, Wiley 2010.

Lourie, B & Smith, R. *Toxin Toxout: Getting Harmful Chemicals Out of Our Bodies and Our World*, St. Martin's Griffin, 2015.

Maizes, V. *Be Fruitful: The Essential Guide to Maximizing Fertility and Giving Birth to a Healthy Child*, Scribner, 2013.

Pizzorno, J. *The Toxin Solution: How Hidden Poisons in the Air, Water, Food, and Products We Use Are Destroying Our Health--AND WHAT WE CAN DO TO FIX IT*, Harper One, 2018.

Simon, D & Chopra, D. *The Wisdom of Healing: A Natural Mind Body Program for Optimal Wellness*, Harmony, 1998.

Smith, R & Lourie, B. *Slow Death by Rubber Duck: The Secret Danger of Everyday Things*, Counterpoint, 2011.

Acknowledgements

I have immense gratitude for everyone involved in my journey to create this book. Many teachers inspired me with their wisdom and their work. My biggest thanks goes to Dr. Deepak Chopra, from whom I began to learn more than twenty-five years ago. He paved the way for physicians like me to integrate Western allopathic medicine with other healing modalities and, together with Dr. David Simon, co-founded the Chopra Center for Wellbeing where they brought Ayurvedic practices including "detox" into the modern day. In particular, their work in mind-body medicine and spirituality has opened the discussion of compassion, meditation, and mindfulness in health and wellness to a larger audience, including the scientific community. It was with their guidance that I was able to heal and transform myself and then became inspired to help others do the same. Working closely with Dr. Simon, I learned so much about life, death, and the art of medicine.

I have been blessed with so many other wonderful teachers guiding me on my path, including Drs. Robert Bonakdar, Joseph Helms, Mimi Guarneri, James Gordon, Mark Hyman, Jenny Quintana, Andrew Weil, Tieraona Low Dog, Victoria Maizes, Anjali Sharma, Rajesh Sharma, Jeff Bland, Bob Rountree, and Walter Crinnion; instructors at the Center for Mind Body Medicine, the University of Arizona Center for Integrative Medicine (and thanks to the Bravewell Collaborative and Dr. Ellen Beck for making this part of my education possible), and the Institute for Functional Medicine; colleagues at Scripps Center for Integrative Medicine including Drs. David

Leopold, Raneth Heng, and Chris Suhar, Rauni King, Brenda Rodi, Karen Sothers, Fay McGrew, and Liz Fraser; and Chopra Center educators Davidji and Drs. Suhas Kshirsagar, David Frawley, and Dan Vicario.

I am grateful for the patients and guests at the Chopra Center for Wellbeing, with and for whom I have studied. It is through my quest to find the answers for their health issues that I discovered that I needed to go beyond what I had learned, to go beyond what we were already doing, and to evolve to a new way of practicing medicine.

In the midst of writing this book, I faced my own health challenge and I am so thankful for the staff at the Chopra Center and Mind-Body Medical Group who supported me during my time of healing. I am particularly grateful for Dr. Sheila Patel, whose patience and compassion is unparalleled.

Without the help of a few friends, it would have taken a lot longer to get this book actually written and more than just an idea. Thanks to Maureen Pisani, Patricia McElroy, Carolyn Rangel, Dr. Mona Saint, and Ruth Westreich for your encouragement and enthusiasm. Thanks also to my team at Trident Media: Amanda Annis, Nicole Robson, and Caitlin O'Beirne.

Most of all, I am so thankful for my family for their loving support: my parents, John and Kay Booth, who nurtured my inquisitive spirit; my children, Grace and Annika, who bring me such joy and laughter and also bring out the mama bear in me to protect them and all of the beings in this world; my extended family, who have taken care of the kids, me, fed us, and kept the house running including Jan and George Porter, Becky Smith, and Jeanie Berglund; my sisters, Evelyn and Susan, who provided editorial guidance, humor, and cheered me on; and my husband, Greg, who has stood by me through it all with love and positivity.

About the Author

Dr. Valencia Porter is a leader in Integrative, Holistic, Environmental, and Preventive Medicine who inspires and informs people to live their best lives. Passionate about nutrition, she believes that eating healthy and delicious foods is at the core of our state of health. She has a deep concern for the environment, acknowledging that our health and the health of our planet are intricately linked. In helping her patients find answers to chronic and unexplained conditions, Dr. Porter has studied the effects of environmental toxicants and methods of detoxification as well as why certain people seem to be more susceptible to these effects than others. Her work in this area deepened even further when she was faced with her own health crisis, forcing her to confront her own toxic body burden and inability to detoxify effectively. Digging deep into her healing knowledge, she addressed all layers of mind, body, spirit, and environment to support her body's ability to heal itself from chronic infection, heavy metal toxicity, nutrient depletion, hormonal imbalances, food sensitivities, neurologic impairment, and chronic pain. Dr. Porter believes that medical care should be personalized and that treatment plans need to be tailored to the individual in partnership rather than set in a standard protocol. She also recognizes that our mental and emotional states greatly affect our health and has led many patients from a state of chronic stress and disease to leading a more balanced, vibrant, and joyful life.

For the last decade, Dr. Porter has worked with Dr. Deepak Chopra at the Chopra Center for Wellbeing, where she provides integrative medical consultations and teaches both health professionals and the community. She combines the best of conventional medicine and complementary modalities to help individuals achieve their health and wellness goals utilizing her knowledge of Ayurveda, yoga, meditation, functional medicine, environmental medicine, nutrition, herbal medicine, and other healing traditions. At the Chopra Center, she served in various positions including Director of Women's Health, Director of Integrative Medicine, and Medical Director. She is also part of the Chopra Center research team, which is looking at the effects of meditation, yoga, and Ayurvedic practices on health outcomes. In addition to her work at the Chopra Center, Dr. Porter has a private consulting and coaching practice.

After studying Computer Science and Cognitive Science at Tufts University, Dr. Porter received her medical degree from the University of Southern California and completed a residency in General Preventive Medicine at the University of California San Diego. She then completed a Fellowship in Integrative Medicine at the University of Arizona where she was a Bravewell Collaborative scholar. Double board-certified, she was one of the first physicians to achieve board certification in Integrative Medicine and serves on the American Board of Integrative Medicine. Dr. Porter also earned a Master's Degree in Public Health focusing on Environmental Health from San Diego State University, and is on the Steering Committee of the Medical Society Consortium on Climate and Health. A Fellow of the American College of Nutrition, she serves on the Professional Advisory Board of the American Nutrition Association. Dr. Porter has extensive training in many healing modalities and was recently named as one of the "100 Trailblazers in Yoga and Ayurveda" by *Spirituality and Health* magazine.

A sought-after speaker, she engages small groups to audiences greater than 500 attendees. Dr. Porter also enjoys sharing her experience with other healthcare providers and is guest faculty at the Arizona Center for Integrative Medicine, voluntary faculty at the University of California San Diego Department of Family and Preventive Medicine, and a frequent lecturer at Continuing Medical Education seminars. She has published numerous scientific and popular articles and book chapters and is currently working on several books.

She lives in Southern California with her husband and two children and enjoys organic gardening, hiking, yoga, reading books in print, and the performing arts.

Connect with Valencia Porter Online:

Facebook: www.facebook.com/VPorterMD/
Twitter: twitter.com/VPorterMD
Blog: valenciaporter.com/blog/
Website: valenciaporter.com

CPSIA information can be obtained
at www.ICGtesting.com
Printed in the USA
LVHW052030101218
599931LV00025B/1735